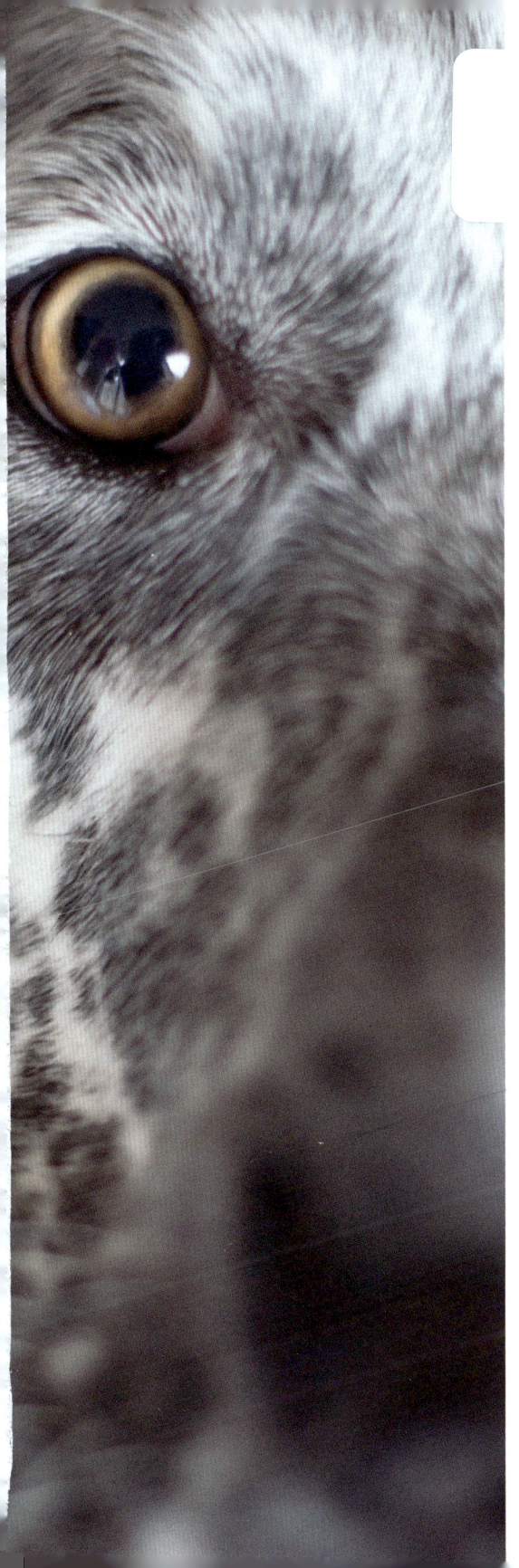

Eat Your Own Dog Food Series

Say **"No"** to DOG FOOD!

Dine With Your Best Friend...
Share Healthful Meals Using
the
4-PAWS-PLUS Plan™

By Luna Lindbergh
with Lori Lindbergh

Eat Your Own Dog Food Series

"If you want to lead an extraordinary life, find out what the ordinary do—and don't do it."

-Author, Tommy Newberry

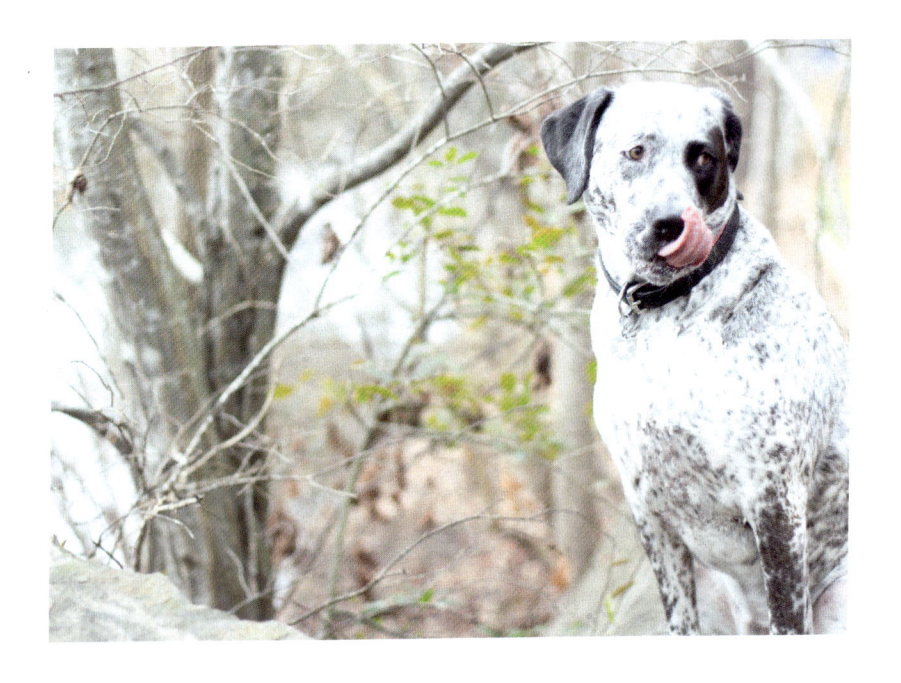

Eat Your Own Dog Food Series

Acknowledgments

Thank you mom and dad for truly treating me like a member of your family and letting me share your lives; we have become quite the inseparable pack. And thank you Kristin and Scott Tyson at SBT Imaging, my sister and brother-in-law, for editing my manuscript and taking such awesome photographs of me enjoying my life. I have a great life! Finally, a huge thank you to Jennifer Feaster, my cousin and artistic designer, for creating our cool logo. Her design has captured the tail-wagging, fun-loving, whimsical nature of my life and the Eat Your Own Dog Food Series of books.

Copyright © Lori Lindbergh 2014. All rights reserved.

No part of this book may be used or reproduced by any means, graphic, electronic, or mechanical, including photocopying, recording, or by any information storage retrieval system without the written permission of the author except in the case of brief quotations embodied in critical articles and reviews.

ISBN: 978-0-9915859-0-8

The Blurb-provided layout designs and graphic elements are copyright Blurb Inc. This book was created using the Blurb creative publishing service. The book author retains sole copyright to his or her contributions to this book.

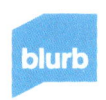

Contents

Think Out of the Bag...Are You Ready to Get that Smelly, Brown Kibble **OUT** of Your Bowl?	6
Meet My Mom	8
Eating the Same Thing Every Day...How Boring is That?	12
What is Real Food? Look at the Picture on the Dog Food Bag, Not Inside the Bag	16
Make the Transition Carefully and Thoughtfully	18
You are What You Eat. Are You Off the Chart?	20
You Need The Right Tools for the Job	22
The Well-Stocked Pantry, Refrigerator, & Freezer	26
Now What? It's as Easy as 1, 2, 3, 4: The **4-PAWS-PLUS Plan**™	28
Almost Ready for Great Eating...No Supersizing Allowed	32
4-PAWS-PLUS Plan™ Ten Basic Guidelines	38
Main ARF-Fair	42
Vege-TAILbles & Flanks	84
Nibbles & PAW-Food	98
InDOGences	114
Special Theme-Day ARF-Fairs	132
Appendix A: Pantry, Refrigerator, & Freezer Inventory	134
Appendix B: Other Tips & Suggestions	137

Eat Your Own Dog Food Series

Think Out of the Bag...Are You Ready to Get that Smelly, Brown Kibble OUT of Your Bowl?

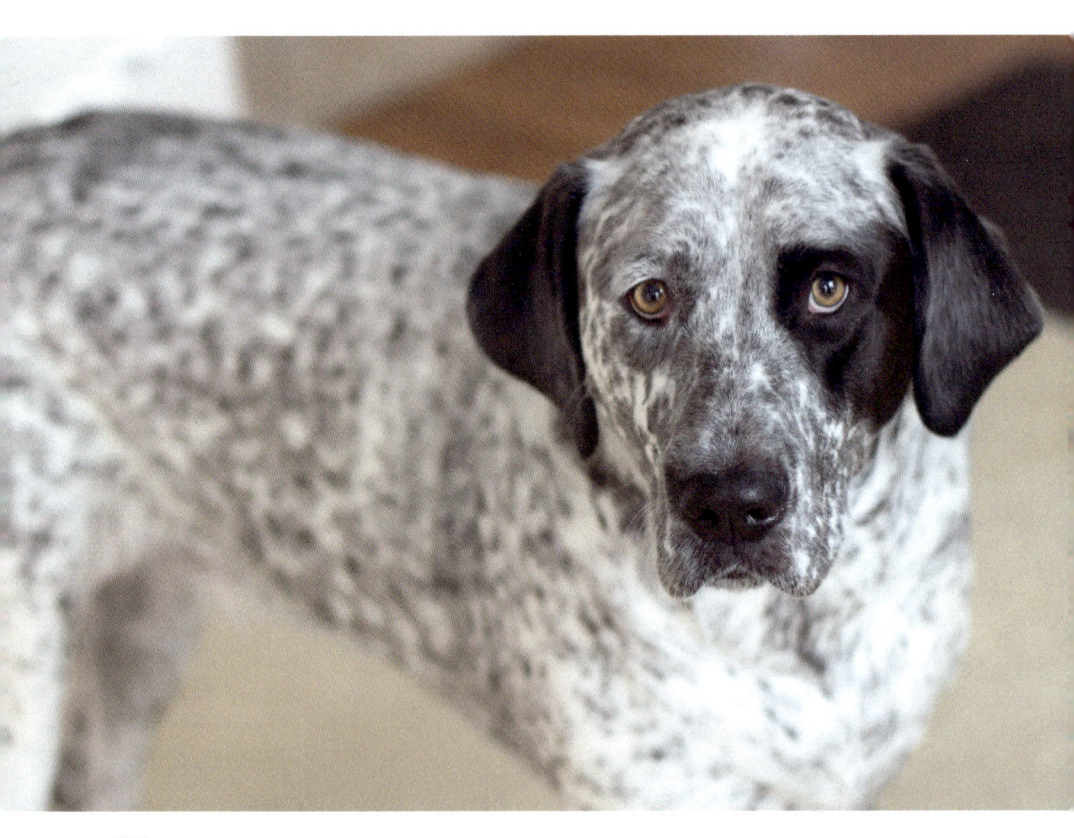

Hello, my name is **Luna**.

I am a 100-pound Labrador retriever mixed breed born on May 7, 2011. That is what the Guilford County Animal Shelter in Greensboro, NC told my mom and dad when they adopted me. I was 4-months old and weighed only 25-pounds when they brought me home. For the past two years, my mom has been feeding me **"real food," not dog food**. She says, "There is no such thing as dog food or people food; there's just food, some food more nutritious than other food."

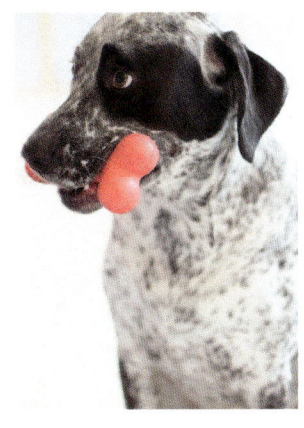

At my house, we dine together as a family every day eating healthful meals. You too can do the same at your house.

This book will help your moms and dads just **Say "NO" to Dog Food**.

My mom says that *Eat Your Own Dog Food* is a phrase that means to use one's own product or service. I wonder how many dog parents who work at dog food factories use their own products, literally.

They may feed their products to their own dogs; however, if this healthy and holistic dog food is "made from the finest natural ingredients so you can love your dog like family, and feed your dog like family," why not serve a tasty plate of kibble lasagna or all-natural, organic kibble stew to the whole family for dinner? Yuck, that's what I thought.

This book will help your parents, who may reluctantly, yet faithfully scoop brown, smelly kibble into your bowls every day, wondering and wishing that they had something better to feed you. Well, I am here to show you that they do, and we do notice the difference. If your parents like to cook and are looking for a reason to enjoy cooking, have them look no further. Here is their opportunity to cook healthful meals and dine with you, their canine best friend (or all of their best friends). How cool is that?

Your parents can use this book to enjoy an occasional meal together with you and they can join my mom's online community at **www.eatyourowndogfood.net** to learn how to get rid of dog food permanently and share healthful meals together every day.

Either way, get ready to chow down on some "really good, real food."

Luna

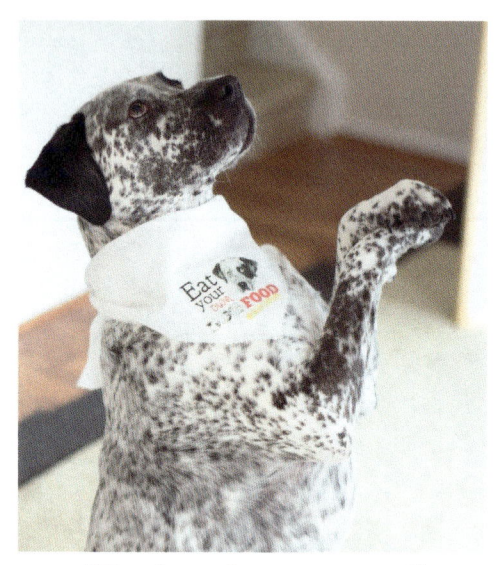

"Thank you for my mommy!"

Meet My Mom

> *"My mom is the best. She is creative and nontraditional and has always questioned mainstream thinking. Lucky for me, and I hope for you, she questioned the automatic belief that dogs must eat dog food."*

My mom started feeding me real food when I was about 10 months old. No, she's not a veterinarian or a nutritionist, just a PhD who knows how to fully review the literature, objectively evaluate science and research, test assumptions, and think critically, to synthesize her findings into relevant, effective actions. Whew, just the sound of that wears me out. (BTW, she is also a licensed registered nurse.)

She practices what she preaches (and dad too): Eating healthful, balanced meals every day and staying flexible and active physically and mentally.

My mom has read many of the nutrition textbooks used in veterinary schools, including the *Nutrient Requirements of Dogs and Cats* by the National Research Council and has used other pet nutrition and diet books (raw diet, ancestral diet, etc.) written by veterinarians and nutritionists. She has assimilated all of this information into her **4-PAWS-PLUS Plan (4-P3)**, so your entire family and you can eat the same healthful meals every day.

There is no need for your mom to make special bulk "dog food" preparations, no need to go all organic or frou-frou (but you can if you want to), and most importantly, no need to be a chef. All she needs to do is use the freshest ingredients that fit within your family's budget and love to cook, or at least have a strong desire to cook or learn how to cook. The fresh meals she will prepare using this book, will no doubt be superior to any processed, packaged dog food you've been eating.

My mom suggests your parents start by taking smaller steps at first to learn the basics, see the results, and then jump in full speed. My mom was a little fearful at first because the industry wants your parents to think dog nutrition is a lot more complicated than human nutrition and that feeding dogs fresh, real food will lead to nutrient imbalances and diseases. After her initial fear and the normal "I don't know what I am doing" feeling passed, my mom jumped in full speed, and she hasn't looked back.

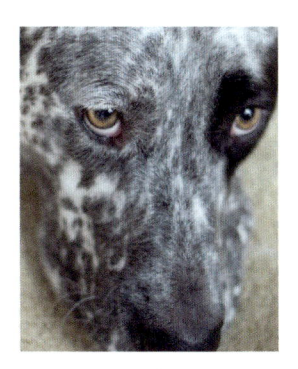

My sneaky look.

I now eat way better than just about any dog I know and most humans too.

My mom has refined her approach over the past two years and has created her easy to use **4-P3** framework to help your parents prepare healthful meals to feed everyone in your household "like family." I continue to be her test subject, but now the rest of our family has joined in. We have eaten some great tasting, nutritious meals, snacks, and desserts (and some not so great ones too, sorry mom).

The rule is that both dad and I must give the one thumb/paw up before a recipe is approved for outside consumption. So here I am, two years later, energetic, strong, and thriving. And I look forward to having dessert every night too, just like most humans do. (Yes, I do know what the word dessert means.)

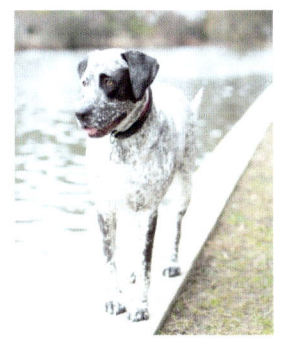

Duck hunting at the neighborhood lake.

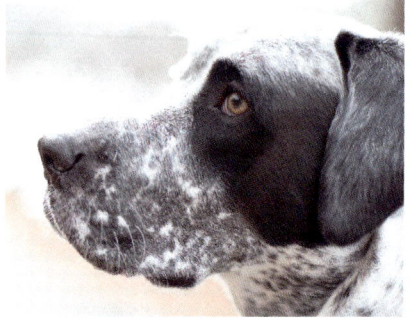

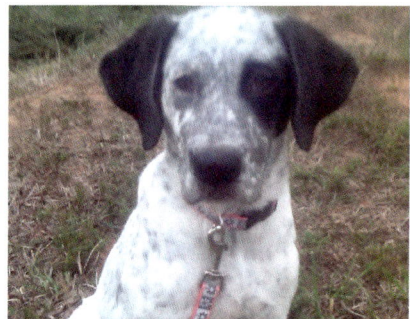

Me, now.   *Me, when mom and dad just brought me home.*

My mom and I have visited a number of different veterinarians because we have traveled quite a bit over the past two years. As expected, every time a new veterinarian asked my mom what she fed me, and my mom said real food, we would get two responses.

The first one, which was the most common, was a look of shock and disbelief, like OMG, are you crazy, how can your dog possibly be getting all the nutrients she needs? Then there was the second response, "I too give my dog human food on occasion," or, "I just made a big pot of dog food for my dog." To that response, my mom always asked, "How was it; did you eat it too?" The response to that was a strange look on their faces and, "Oh no, it's dog food."

With the help of my mom (and my dad who won't let me become a couch PAW-tato), I am living proof that dogs can thrive and stay fully nourished (with minimal supplements) eating the same meals that humans eat every day. However, I do have a few additional nutrient requirements (as you will see later) and must avoid certain foods all together. But that doesn't mean your parents need to give up those foods. My mom has done the hard work and will show you how everything fits together in her easy to use plan; all you have to do now is have fun and enjoy the dining experience.

Thanks Mom!

Eat Your Own Dog Food Series

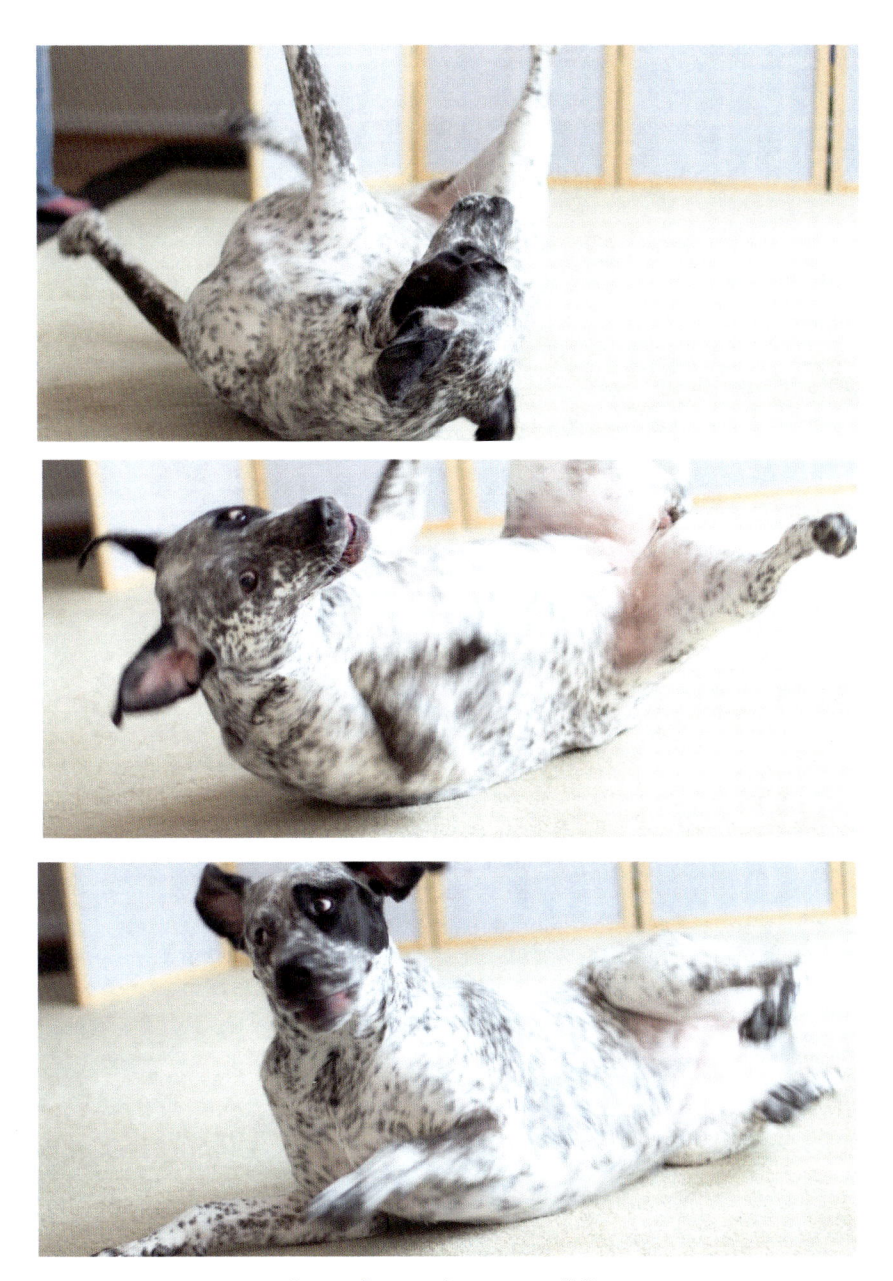

"Watch out, I'm on a roll."

Meet My Mom 11

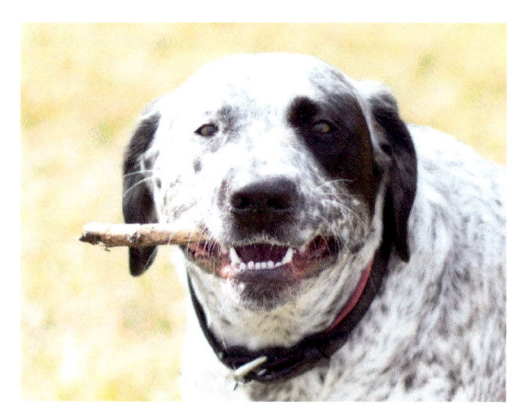

"Still, nothin' beats a good after-dinner stick!"

Eating the Same Thing Every Day...How Boring is That?

"What do you think your mom and dad would say if they had no choice but to eat the same irresistible, fake chicken- or beef-smelling, brown kibble every day? They probably would think that was pretty boring too."

Have you ever heard your parents say things, such as, "You are just a dog; dogs don't know the difference; dogs don't care what they eat; it doesn't make any difference what a dog eats."

I am here to say, with the help of my mom and dad of course, that from my perspective, your parents are wrong. It does matter what I eat, and I do know the difference between dog food and real, nutritious meals. And most importantly, my body knows the difference too.

Eating the same dog food every day should seem dull to us dogs; however, the strong artificial flavorings that are purposefully added to dog food drive us wild; we can't help ourselves.

It's like human junk food with all of the enticing salt, fat, sugar, and additives, but for dogs. Just like many humans who can't resist junk food, we will gulp down our dog food quickly and often overeat, again just like humans.

When my mom started feeding me real food, I wanted to eat all the time. I was still growing and needed to replenish all of the nutritional deficiencies I had from eating dog food. My weight surged (in a good way), and the frequent gastrointestinal irregularity I experienced from eating one of the "best brands" of processed dog food resolved completely.

Dog food always passed through my gut so quickly. When I was 9-months old, I was diagnosed with bilious vomiting syndrome. My veterinarian wanted my mom to give me medication to "slow things down!" My mom questioned that and decided it was time to find a better way. Who knew all I needed to do was stop eating dog food and start eating more healthful, fresh meals.

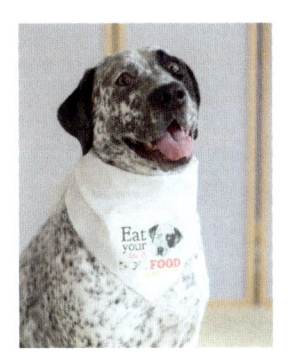

"Say YES to real food!"

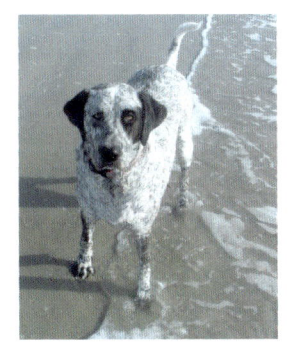

"I love the beach!"

Hmmm, there is a reason veterinarians often recommend human food when dogs are not feeling well.

One and a half years later, I eat only when I'm hungry. Food doesn't drive me wild anymore (except for sardines and desserts). It's more like I drive my mom crazy sometimes because, when I don't get much activity that morning, I don't want to eat until later in the day, even though she serves me a great meal. It makes sense that if I haven't been very active that day, I don't want to eat as much, a behavior most humans should adopt.

I've lost all my puppy fat and am now a muscular, active, well-nourished adult dog. My digestive system and immune system have matured so I can eat just about anything, including corn, dairy, and grains, in moderation, of course. There are a few exceptions noted later that my mom never lets me eat.

Here are some of my favorite meals and snacks—Yes, I really do get to eat these!

MEALS

- Beef Stew
- Chicken Pot Pie
- Pulled Pork Sandwich
- Mom's Homemade Pizza
- Tuna Casserole
- Goat Cheese Frittata
- Spaghetti with Meat Sauce
- Three-Bean Chili
- Chicken Fettuccine Alfredo
- Edamame and Squash Quiche
- Fish Chowder
- Honey Mustard Chicken
- Spinach and Pasta Soup

SNACKS & DESSERTS

- Lemon Apricot Quinoa Muffins
- Peanut Butter Hummus
- Brown Rice and Flax Waffles
- Pear and Apple Galette
- Whipped Cream
- Coconut Macaroons
- Strawberry Custard Tart
- Blueberry Yogurt Cake
- Carrot Cake
- Banana Custard Pie
- White Popcorn
- Peanut Butter Yonannas™
- Quinoa Meatballs

No dog food on this list. Your transformation to eating the foods on this list could be easy because your mom may already be cooking for the rest of your family. My mom says that eliminating dog food may cost a little more, depending on your size and the brand of dog food you have been eating, but won't add much more time to her regular cooking schedule. Also, your parents will never run out of dog food, so this will eliminate all those trips to the dog food store.

Cooking for you requires a little more thinking than simply tearing open a bag of dog food or opening up a can and dumping it into your bowl. However, when your parents see the changes in your behavior and the calming effect you experience from eating satisfying, real food; plus, when they experience the joy of dining together as a family, they will agree the time, effort, and thinking are well worth it. Not to mention the health benefits they may experience from eating less junk food, reducing their salt intake, and eliminating sugar, preservatives, and all prepackaged foods from their diets.

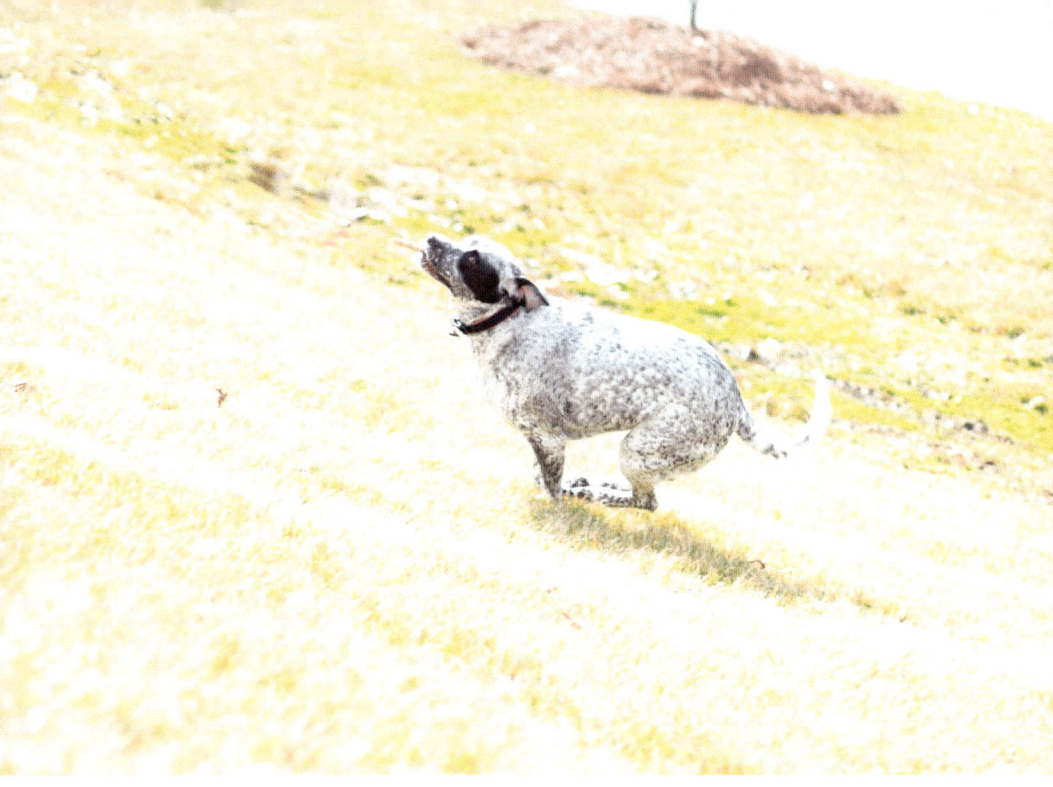

"Full of energy, not junk food."

If your parents are reading this book, they must already think of you as more than just a "dog" anyway, so they can view the cost and effort as being similar to feeding a new small child; however, in my case I eat more like a large adult child.

This is simply another way your parents can truly love you like family! They can even get the whole family involved in the transformation.

One last thing. Please be sure to warn your parents that you might lose your taste for dog food once you experience eating real, fresh, wholesome food.

Time to chow down!

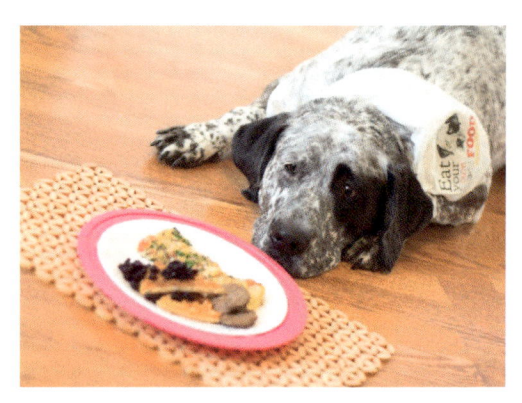

"Eggs, waffles with blueberries, and sausage, my favorite, but I say that about everything mom makes!"

What is Real Food? Look at the Picture on the Dog Food Bag, Not Inside the Bag

"If you want to know what real food looks like, look at the picture on the dog food bag, not what's inside the bag. Whuff, my chicken and beef don't look like that!"

No prepackaged, preservative-laden, or fast food in our house.

My mom told me when she was growing up, her mother fed the family dog Taffy, a small mixed terrier, various canned and bagged dog food and yummy processed, fake-flavored dog treats. That's just what you did back then, and that's just what your parents think they need to do now.

After a while, in addition to dog food, everyone in my mom's family began feeding Taffy table scraps, caffeinated coffee beverages with cream and sugar, hamburger helper, hot dogs, cookies, cakes, and just about anything else the family happened to be eating that day (except chocolate).

Needless to say, Taffy became obese and eventually developed insulin-dependent diabetes, thus supporting the pet food industry's claims (and most veterinarians): Dogs should eat dog food only, and giving a dog "human food" will make a dog obese. Seriously?? Too much food of any kind will lead to overweight dogs and overweight humans.

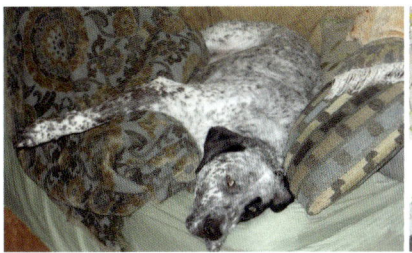

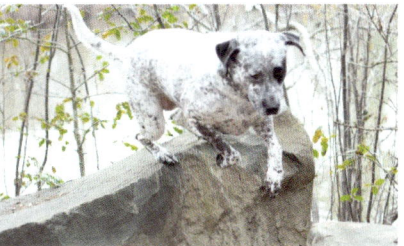

"From couch PAW-tato to outdoor adventurer in 2 seconds flat!"

What my mom means by real food is that chicken looks like chicken, carrots and sweet potatoes look like carrots and sweet potatoes, and blueberries look like blueberries, because they are, and they are not just photos on the bag. My mom cooks and bakes most everything from scratch. We do not eat granulated white or brown sugar, artificial sweeteners, white flour, high fructose corn syrup, evaporated cane juice, salt, hydrogenated oils, or the natural flavorings and preservatives found in most prepared foods. If a food label lists more than four or five ingredients, my mom stops reading and puts it back on the shelf.

She buys milk, eggs, and good quality lean meats with minimal additives from the local warehouse store or grocery store, and buys organic, grass-fed, or free-range meat, poultry, and eggs when available. We eat fish once or twice a week, in addition to the sardines dad and I share, and often mom includes a vegetarian meal each week. Dad hates that; he is a true carnivore, like me.

We eat lots of fruits and vegetables, some organic, most not however, and minimal canned goods. I like to eat some fruits raw, such as bananas, oranges, and cherries; however, most of the fruits and vegetables I eat are incorporated into my meals. I like all fruits and vegetables in my meals, but don't like to eat many of them raw or plain any longer. When all is said and done, my parents eat what I eat, and I eat what they eat because there is no such thing as dog food; however, as you will see in the next section, there are a few things that my mom NEVER feeds me.

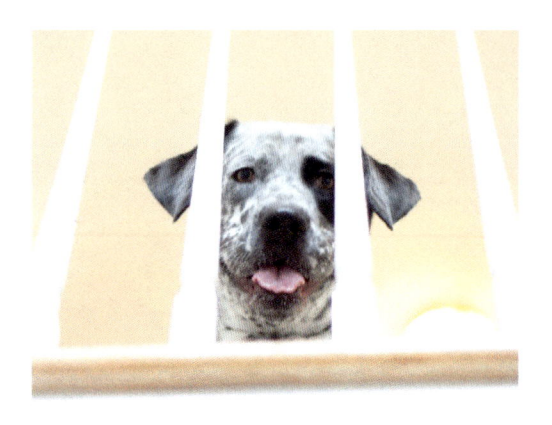

*"Time to break outta the **Dog Food Rut**!"*

Make the Transition Carefully and Thoughtfully

"The most important things your parents need to know are that there are specific foods that they should never feed you and that portion control is the key."

I started eating only real food when I was about 10 months old. Prior to that, my mom had been supplementing my processed, bagged dog food with green beans, carrots, and pumpkin as recommended by my veterinarian and trainer to help relieve my hunger pangs, diarrhea, and periodic morning vomiting. I wanted to eat grass all the time too.

Even though my digestive system may have been a little immature, I tolerated the switch to real food immediately. Within a couple of weeks, my gastrointestinal symptoms resolved, and I stopped wanting to eat grass. I was calm and satisfied.

Most veterinarians who believe in real food diets for dogs recommend using a slow transition from dog food to real food and suggest trying out different foods to see what you like or don't like. Mom made the switch, cold turkey. (Yum, I like that too.) She started out using several "dog food cookbooks" for making the typical homemade dog food mixes that only I was supposed to eat. She finally got tired of cooking different food for me and cooking regular meals for dad and herself. It didn't make sense; she was using the same fresh ingredients for both of us, but spending extra effort making two different meals.

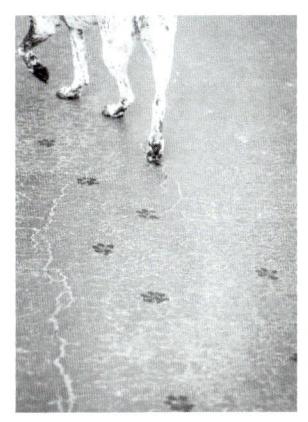

That is when she decided to figure out how to cook one meal for all of us to eat. After a few adjustments, we all eat the same meals now. I can eat most everything, but some foods in lesser amounts. You will see this in each recipe where I offer my tips and suggestions to help you with portions.

My mom recommends this book for parents of relatively healthy, active dogs and for dogs like me who can't seem to tolerate any type of processed dog food.

However, this book may be helpful for parents of dogs with known diseases, dietary restrictions, or known food allergies. With a real food diet, it is very easy for your mom and dad to eliminate the food item(s) causing your allergy or problem. You can't really do that with most dog foods because, "it is what it is." (That's what dad always says.)

One difference is that unlike dog food with easy measuring instructions on the label, with real food, it is very easy for your mom and dad to be a bit more generous in your portions, so they need to be more mindful when sizing your portions. Just as many humans do, you too could become overweight or obese from eating too much real food, which again supports the dog food industry's claim that giving real food to dogs leads to obesity. However, I've seen a lot of overweight dog-food dogs too. Mom says that food does not lead to obesity, poor eating habits and reduced activity levels lead to obesity.

Here is a list of foods your mom and dad should **NOT** feed you. There are a number of web sites on the internet that provide more details on why these should be avoided.

MOM'S DO NOT FEED ME LIST

Chocolate	Candy	Onions
Macadamia Nuts	Gum	Garlic
Grapes	Cooked Bones	Avocados
Raisins	Excessive Salt	Alcohol
Coffee, Tea, Caffeine	Artificial Sweeteners	Refined Sugars

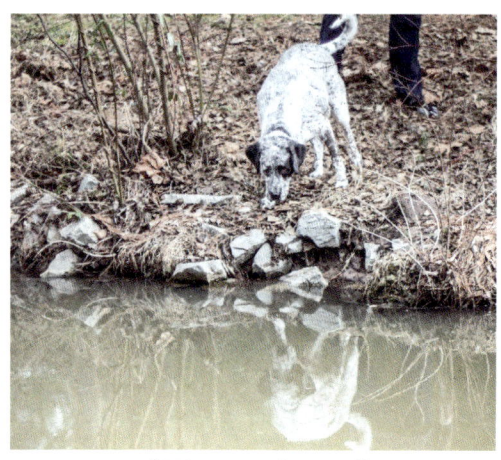

"Mirror, mirror..."

You Are What You Eat. Are You Off the Chart?

"I meet many dog friends on my daily walks. No matter where I go, I hear their parents offer comments about me to my parents, such as, "What a beautiful dog, what a big dog, she looks so strong, and she is so soft."

Well, I'm here to tell you, that the reason my parents hear these comments is because, "I am what I eat." And I am lucky that I can eat any type of real food, including grains, corn, gluten-free, vegan, and dairy; all in moderation, of course. The reason I can eat all of these foods is because my mom does not feed me the same thing every day. She strives for weekly nutritional balance using a variety of foods.

I'm no size-zero, runway-model dog, nor am I an undernourished dog-food-weight-chart dog. However, I'm no overweight couch PAW-tato either. In fact, the body style created by my breed combination doesn't seem to fit on the "ideal-dog" weight chart, which BTW was most likely created for average dog-food dogs.

From his research, my dad thinks I have many of the characteristics of a Blue Gascon hound, especially the coloring of my coat and size and shape of my tail. These characteristics combined with those of a Labrador retriever create a naturally thick and extra-long torso. I have a large, deep chest that curves into my stomach rather than having that extreme tucked up look and tapered waist. He also found that I have the potential to weigh up to 110 pounds!

Eat Your Own Dog Food Series

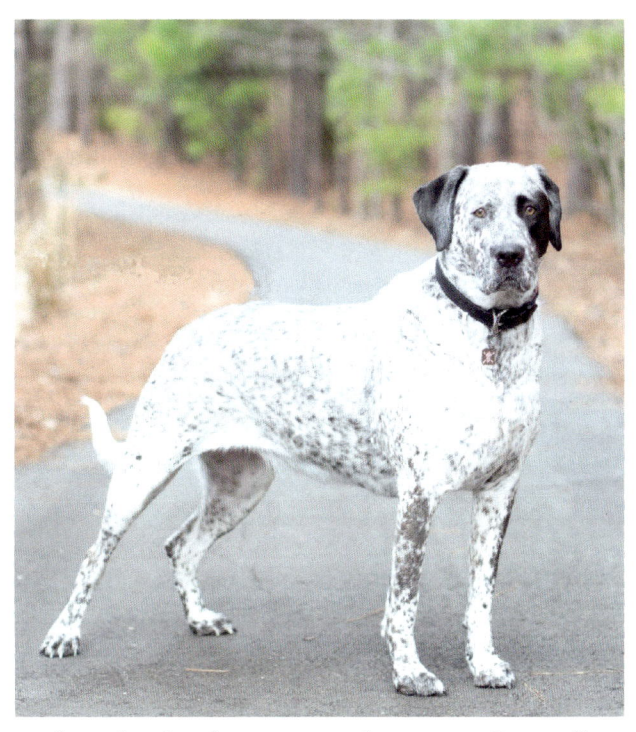

"Go ahead, I dare you....to be extraordinary!"

Even as a skinny little puppy from the shelter, my mom said I had a thick torso and never had a small tapered waist like you see on the weight chart. And I've always had my loose hanging "jelly belly" as mom calls it.

I walk and run 3 or more miles per day, jump, tug, sniff, and play many times a day, and have great energy. I would play all day if dad would oblige my every request. I'm just a big dog with a well-nourished body and a thick skin and coat, thanks to the nutritious meals my mom feeds me everyday. Would you call a performance athlete or body builder "overweight?" Similar to human body composition, there are exceptions to the rule, outliers from the average, and limitless possibilities.

"It's Time to Think Off the Chart!

You Are What You Eat

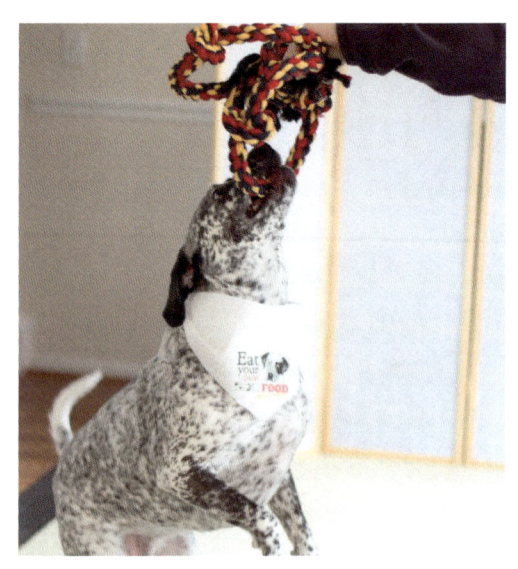

"The toys make all the difference"

You Need the Right Toys for the Job

"My mom sure loves her kitchen toys as much as I like mine. She uses them often to prepare great meals for me... and dad too."

Your mom will need some basic cooking tools and utensils to begin preparing meals for your entire family. She probably has most of them. Typical things like pots and pans, nonstick skillets, roasting pans, stock pots, microwave cookware, cutting boards, knives for chopping, various-sized metal bowls, and mixing spoons are essential.

My mom always makes enough food for plenty of leftovers so a set of small freezer- and microwave-safe containers will be helpful. She uses these containers to freeze broth, beans, pasta, and rice to use later on. Resealable plastic bags work well for freezing chopped vegetables, breads, muffins and crackers.

Special Toys

If you are a big dog like me and eat a lot, these special toys will help your mom keep up. Your parents can purchase all of these from home stores or online retailers, such as Amazon.

I love when mom orders from Amazon. The UPS driver brings me bubble wrap to pop and play with every time he comes to visit. Here are a few of my mom's favorite special toys.

Electric Pressure Cooker. This is her new favorite. My mom uses this to roast meat, cook rice and beans, and make one-pot meals, soups, and stews. You can find one of these at a home store or online retailer. Think of this as a slow cooker on steroids!

Bread Machine. Any bread machine will do. We eat only homemade bread, rolls, flatbread, and pizza crust. My mom spends only 10-15 minutes throughout the bread-making process adding the ingredients to the machine and shaping the rolls and breads; the machine does the hard part, including the mixing, kneading, and dough rising.

Stick Blender. Mom thinks this is the coolest toy ever. She uses it to purée and mix, plus the one she has includes a small food processor for quick chopping and for making salsa. She says clean-up is a breeze.

Waffle Iron. Any standard waffle iron will do. My favorite brown rice and flax waffles are a snap to make. Mom makes extra and freezes them so I can have a waffle for a quick snack anytime.

Electric Griddle. This is great for making pancakes, fritters, and for making flat bread; although, a larger nonstick skillet or cast iron skillet will work just fine.

Food Processor. My mom is still using the hand-held food slicer she bought back in 1985. They don't make appliances like that anymore. She also has an 8-cup table-top food processor for bigger jobs. A food processor will help you grate carrots, nuts, cheeses, and other foods and make hummus and other puréed foods.

Hand-Held Grater or Mandoline Slicer. For quick grating, my mom uses a hand grater or mandoline instead of the food processor. These can make grating cheese or slicing sweet potatoes for fries much easier.

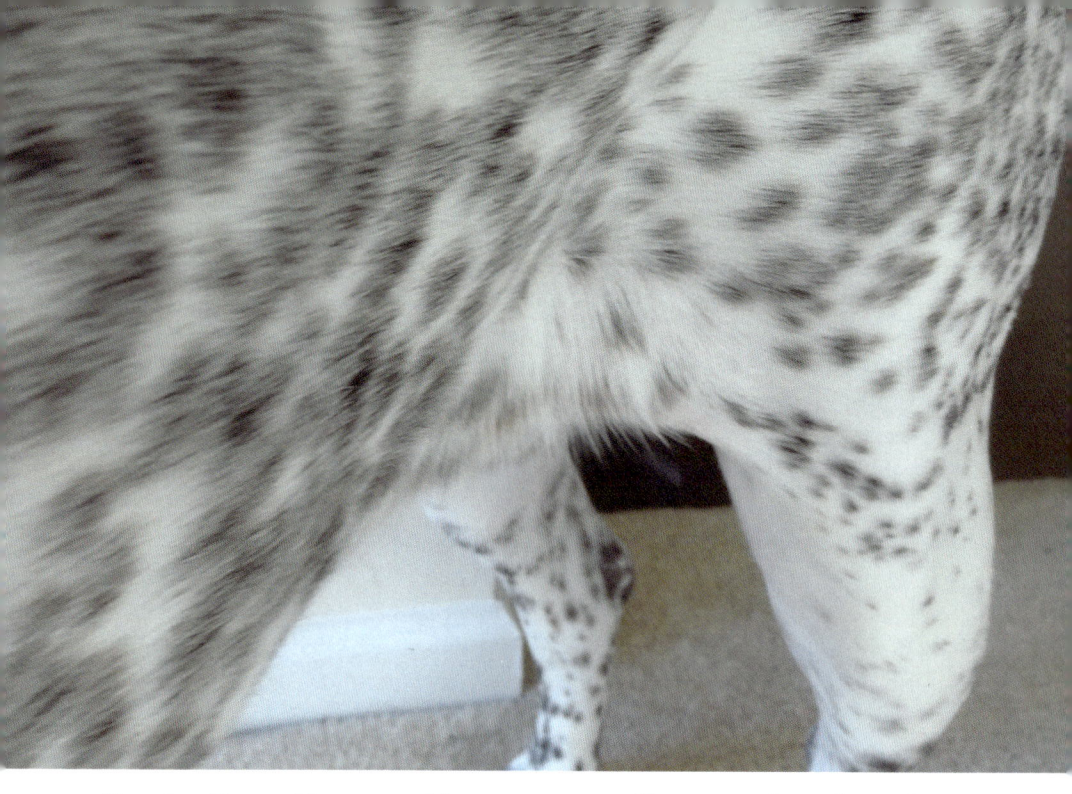

Toaster Oven: Mom uses this to toast my waffles, roast almonds, and reheat pizza and other leftovers.

Spice/Coffee Grinder. This helps with grinding egg shells for my calcium supplement and grinding spices for enhancing the flavor of my meals.

Oil Sprayer. My mom uses one of these for olive oil and canola oil. It helps reduce the amount of oil you need and makes it easier to disperse the oil. She does use canola and olive oil nonstick cooking spray too.

Apple Corer. I love apples, but the seeds are poisonous for me. This helps keep apples safe for me. Mom uses this to remove the center of her cupcakes to insert fresh fruit filling...yum!

Freezer. To save preparation time and have leftovers available for when you don't have time to cook, she recommends your parents invest in a small freezer.

When my mom purchases a new kitchen gadget to help her make new and different great meals, she thinks of it as an investment in the safety, health, and well-being of our family.

Your mom does not have to purchase all of these from the start. She can see what kinds of meals your family members and you like and buy the gadgets that will help her be more efficient in preparing those foods.

My mom says that cooking from scratch requires a bit more effort than buying premade and prepackaged foods, but it does not have to take a lot more time.

Using these gadgets, your parents can finish much of the preparation and chopping for the week's meals ahead of time, to minimize the time they have to spend cooking.

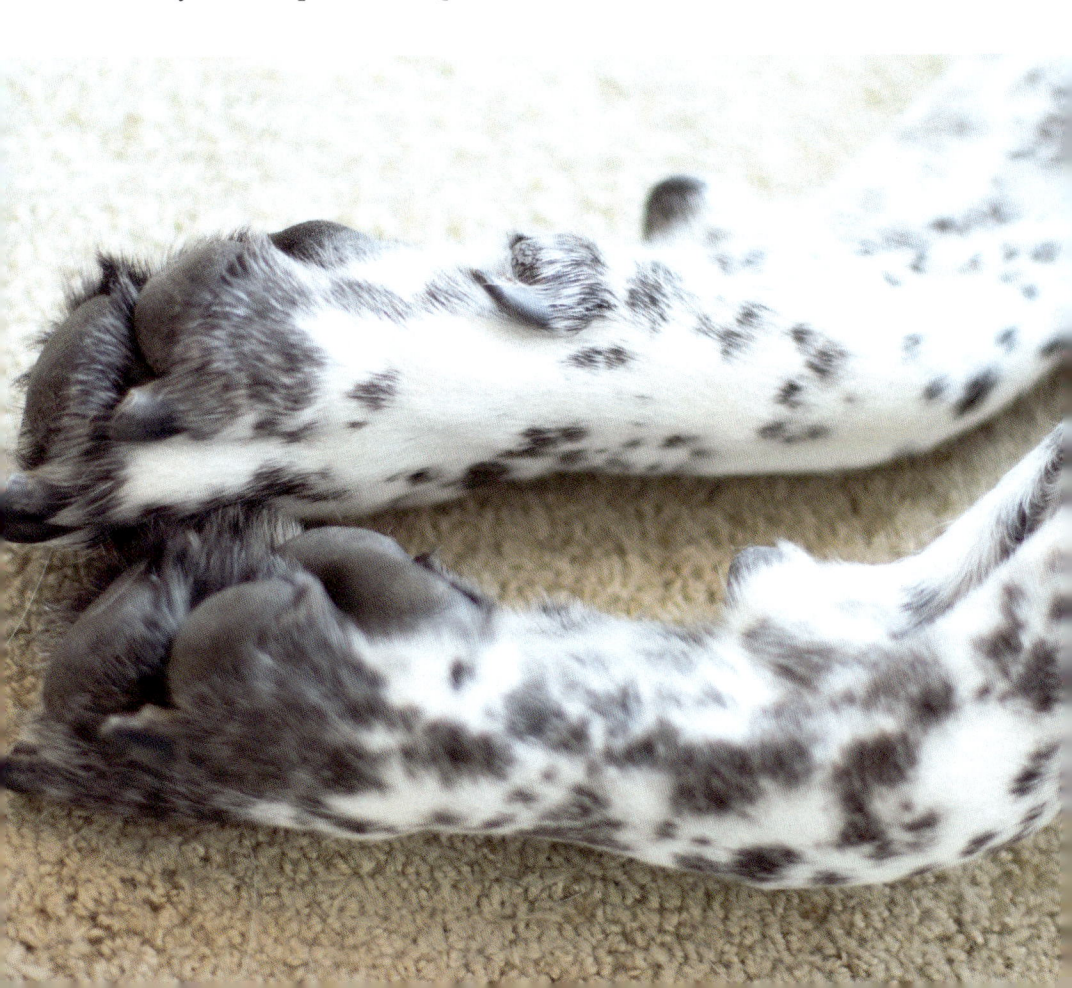

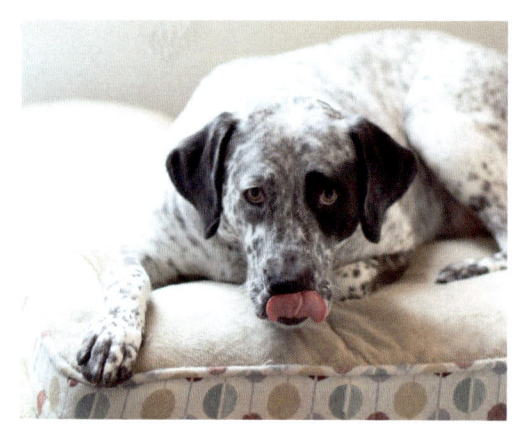

"Yum"

The Well-Stocked Pantry, Refrigerator, & Freezer

"When my mom opens the pantry, refrigerator, or freezer, I get ready to have a great meal. Sometimes I have to wait, but the smell is worth the wait."

My mom says that the key to always being able to cook healthy, flavorful meals, snacks, and desserts is keeping a well-stocked pantry, refrigerator, and freezer. Your mom will now be able to replace the bags of dog food and boxes of dog treats with fresh meats, fruits and vegetables and healthy staples.

In addition to fresh and frozen meats, here is a summary of the items my mom keeps on hand at any given time. (You can find a more detailed list in the Appendix.) Some of the specialty and harder to find items she buys in bulk online from Amazon, Vitacost, or iHerb.

Pantry: Flours & Meals; Rice, Grains, and Pasta; Dried Beans and Legumes; Dried Fruit; Nuts & Seeds; Sweeteners; Oils; Canned Goods (minimal); Sauces & Vinegars; Dry Spices; Baking Products; and Paper Products.

Refrigerator: Fresh Fruits and Vegetables, Milk and Dairy; Cheeses, Fresh Spices, Fruit Juices.

Freezer: Frozen Fruits and Vegetables.

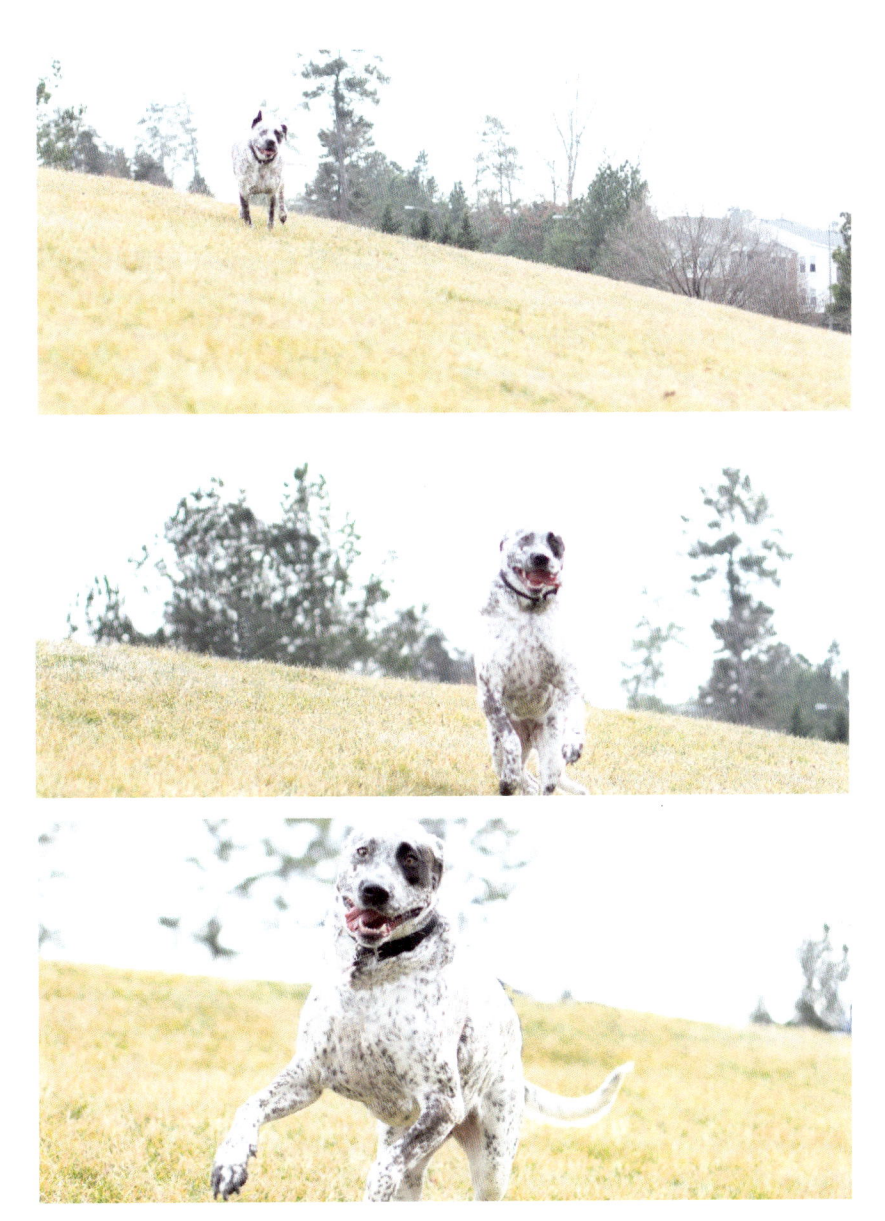

"I love to run, run, run, and run some more!"

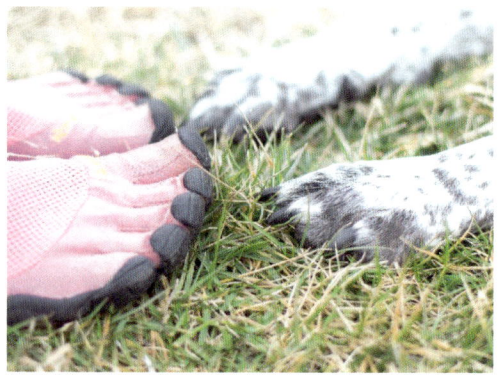

"Look, four paws; Mom has paws too."

Now What? It's as Easy as 1, 2, 3, 4:
The 4-PAWS-PLUS Plan™

*"From her reading and research, my mom has developed the **4-PAWS-PLUS Plan** to help your parents claw their way out of the paper bag, the dog food paper bag, that is!"*

My mom's **4-PAWS-PLUS Plan™ (4-P3)** is an easy to use basic meal framework to help your family and you eat healthful and nutritious meals every day. Here are the major components of her framework.

The **4-PAWS** are:

- **One** Protein (or combination of animal and plant sources)
- **One** Rice, Grain, or Bean
- **Three** or More Vegetables
- **One** Fruit

The **PLUS** adds:

- Additional Protein
- Calcium & Phosphorus (if needed)
- Omega 3s & Omega 6s
- Exercise & Playtime
- Humans Only: Garlic, Onions, Hot Peppers, Salt, & Pepper

Following the **4-P3**™, will help your mom balance the essential nutrients you need each week to stay active, metabolize all of this great food, and help you maintain strong, bones, teeth, muscles, and joints.

I eat twice a day. My mom divides my daily caloric and nutrient requirements into two different tasty meals. Depending on my activity level each day, I eat one or two snacks between meals or one snack during the day and a snack or dessert after dinner. It's hard to resist the cookies and desserts my mom makes! Sometimes she lets me eat dessert first.

My mom has come up with ways to incorporate vegetables and fruits into meals so even finicky humans who don't like vegetables will eat them, sometimes unknowingly. By eating a variety of meats, rice/grains/beans, vegetables, and fruits each week, and my **PLUS** additives every day, I stay well-nourished and energetic.

My mom created the graphic on the next page to depict the **4-PAWS PLUS Plan**™. The graphic is a Venn diagram that consists of four circles, each representing the overlapping **4-PAWS** in the plan.

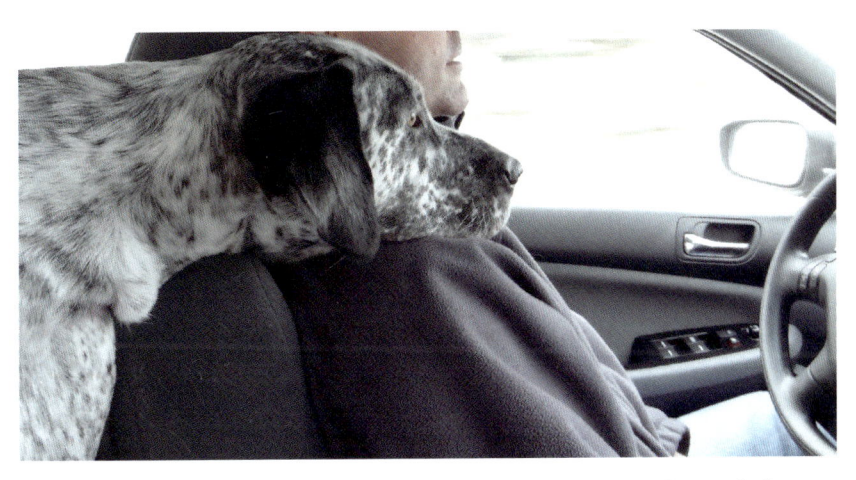

"Cruisin' with dad... I hope we are on our way to the park."

Eat Your Own Dog Food Series

Protein (1)

Rice/ Grain (1)

Fruit (1)

Vegetable (3)

4-PAWS-PLUS Plan™ (4-P3)

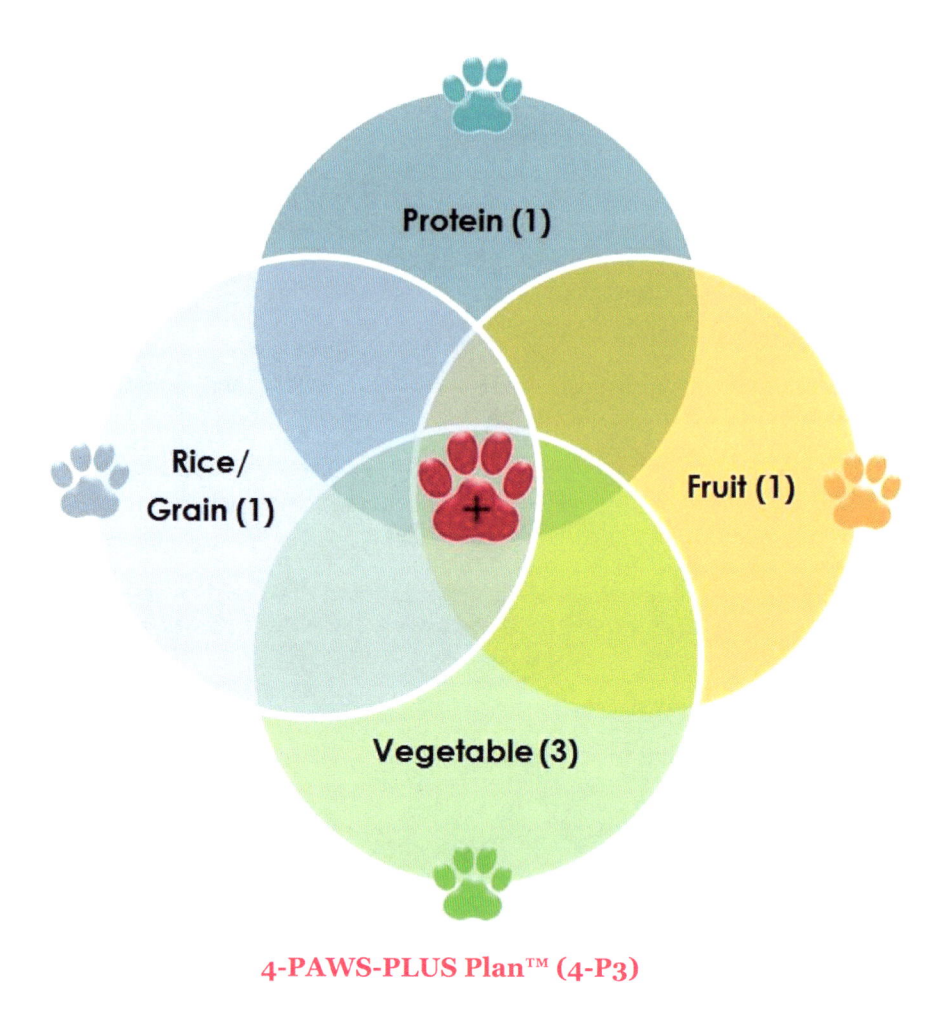

Your mom's goal is to create a meal that hits the center area where all **4-PAWS** overlap, the **Pink PAW**, every day. The closer she comes to achieving that, the more nutritious your meals will be for the day and the overall week.

By mixing up your food components and recipe combinations to achieve the **4-PAWS**, you and your family can share a variety of healthful and nutritious meals, snacks, and desserts. Finally, you don't have to eat the same thing every day or even every week. And don't forget to include the **PLUS** additives; my mom adds these to our meals every day.

Say "NO" to Dog Food

The main meal recipe in this book is marked with the colored **4-PAWS** to show your mom where the recipe fits into the framework and how nutritious the recipe is for you to eat. My mom avoids one-**PAW** foods that are located in only one color of the diagram. She creates complex, nutrient-dense **4-PAW** meals. She says that too many one-**PAW** foods may lead to nutritional imbalances, allergies, and obesity.

For example, my mom's **Meat & Three Bean Chili** is a **4-PAW** meal. It includes all four components:

- **Protein:** beef or chicken and a small amount from the beans.
- **Rice/Grain/Bean**: kidney, pinto, and black beans.
- **Three or More Vegetables**: tomatoes, corn, green peppers, red and yellow peppers, and a few jalapenos.
- **One Fruit**: pear purée (and lime juice).

Here are the **PAW** markings your mom will see to let her know the nutrient components in each recipe.

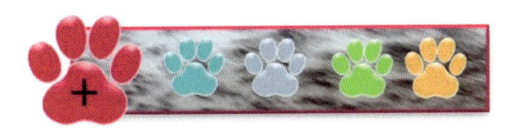

When preparing a recipe that does not have all **4-PAWS**, your mom can add a vegetable, other side, or dessert to balance the meal. When all **4-PAW**S are included, incorporate the additives and suggestions in each recipe next to the **Pink PAW** with the Plus Sign. These suggestions will enhance your meal and create a
more active, healthful, and flavorful dining experience for your family and you.

Your mom can learn how to live the **4-PAWS-PLUS Plan**™ lifestyle by joining my mom's online community of like-minded, health conscious, pet-dining fanatics at **www.eatyourowndogfood.net**. Her weekly recipe subscription program will help your mom completely say,

"NO" to Dog Food.

We can do this together and support each other in making the easy transition to healthful eating and an active lifestyle.

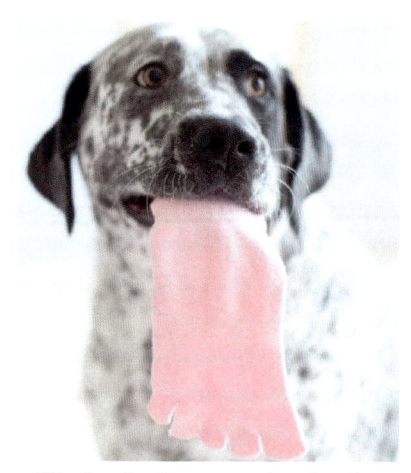

"Socks don't count, they're fat free."

Almost Ready for Great Eating...No Super-Sizing Allowed

"You can always out-eat your exercise! That is why we become overweight. This is where it all comes together and the great eating gets ready to happen!"

Applying the **4-PAWS PLUS Plan**™ is easy once your mom knows how many calories (kilocalories or energy) you expend each day.

All dogs and humans need a certain amount of energy to sustain normal activities in their daily lives. A couch PAW-tato expends less energy than a fitness athlete. However, their energy comes primarily from the same three basic components: Protein, Carbohydrate, and Fat.

My mom compiled the following table using a number of sources, including the National Resource Council's, *Your Dog's Nutritional Needs: A Science-Based Guide for Pet Owners*, to create average daily canine calorie requirements based on your weight.

Remember, these are only averages. If you are more active, less active, or older, you may need to eat more or less per day. This total per day includes calories for all your meals and snacks. Be sure to have your mom check with your veterinarian if she needs more help determining your daily caloric requirements.

Canine Average Daily Caloric Requirements by Body Weight

	\multicolumn{2}{c	}{Small}	\multicolumn{3}{c	}{Medium}
Weight in Pounds	10#	20#	30#	40#	50#
Average Number of Calories Per Day	420	665	945	1,295	1,400

	\multicolumn{3}{c	}{Large}	\multicolumn{2}{c	}{Extra Large}
Weight in Pounds	60#	70#	80#	90#	100#
Average Number of Calories Per Day	1,540	1,820	1,995	2,205	2,450

NOTE: Make sure your mom checks with your veterinarian if she needs to adjust your calorie needs based on increased requirements for pregnancy, lactation, and wound healing.

You can see that naturally, the smaller you are, the fewer calories you need each day. Also, if you are more active one day, your mom can give you a little larger portion that day. My mom has included the portion recommendations on each recipe to balance your daily caloric requirements. **Note: these are just rough estimates to help you adjust your portion sizes.**

The main meals in the **4-PAWS-PLUS Plan™** vary in the percentage of total calories per day derived from the three primary nutrient components.

You (Canine)
- Protein 40-60%
- Carbohydrate 30-50%
- Fat 10-30%

Humans
- Protein 20-50%
- Carbohydrate 30-50%
- Fat 10-30%

Varying the nutrient composition of your meals daily is the key. And, adjusting each meal using the **PLUS** nutritional additives listed on each recipe, will help your mom achieve the canine percentages. Lower fat and carbohydrate options are also suggested for human portions.

Here is a little closer look at each of the **4-PAWS**:

Teal PAW: Protein (and Fat)

The **Teal PAW** sources my mom feeds me include beef, chicken, turkey, pork, liver, eggs and dairy, fish, sardines, beans, and other vegetable sources.

To achieve the **Teal PAW**, the food preparation contains a good protein source for a balance of essential amino acids and fats from organ and muscle meats.

You get much of your daily energy from protein and fat so your requirements for both of these are higher than what humans typically need.

Fat sources include meats and animal products and limited vegetable sources.

Higher Protein and Fat content for your diet compared to humans will be achieved by including the appropriate **PLUS** additives in your meals.

Gray PAW: Rice, Grains, & Beans

The **Gray PAW** sources my mom feeds me include long-grain brown rice, beans, lentils, nuts, quinoa, sweet potatoes, oats, and whole grains breads.

To achieve the **Gray PAW**, the food preparation contains a good source of complex carbohydrates and fiber. Complex, lower-glycemic carbohydrates are a good source of energy and provide vitamins, minerals, and fiber.

Complex carbohydrate intake makes up less of your daily caloric intake compared to humans.

Many recipes use a combination of wheat and gluten-free sources including chick peas, almond flour, arrowroot, soy flour, brown rice flour, amaranth flour, and quinoa and quinoa flour.

Green PAW: Vegetables

The **Green PAW** sources my mom feeds me include kale, escarole, tomatoes, broccoli, carrots, zucchini, green beans, green peppers, red and yellow peppers, spinach, mushrooms, corn, and peas.

To achieve the **Green PAW,** the food preparation contains at least **three** vegetables of varying colors and nutrient content. Vegetables are rich in vitamins, minerals, antioxidants, and fiber.

Vegetables are included in your carbohydrate caloric requirement.

Main meal recipes balance the use low-starchy (e.g., zucchini, greens, cabbage, and peppers) and high-starchy (e.g., butternut squash, peas, and sweet potatoes) vegetables.

Vegetables are cooked into the food to make them easier to digest.

Yellow PAW: Fruits

The **Yellow PAW** sources my mom feeds me include blueberries, strawberries, apples, pears, peaches, apricots, cherries, mixed berries, dates, figs, oranges, and bananas.

To achieve the Yellow PAW, the food preparation contains at least one fruit. Fruits are rich in vitamins, minerals, micronutrients, antioxidants.

Fruits are included in your daily carbohydrate caloric requirement.

Main meal recipes incorporate fruit purées for natural sweetening and include a variety of fruits throughout the week.

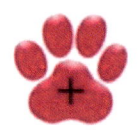

Pink PLUS PAW: Additives

To achieve the **Pink PLUS PAW**, the food preparation contains all of the **4-PAWS**. Prior to serving, your mom should incorporate the PLUS additives listed below to make the experience more complete, flavorful, and fun. These include

Additives For You:

- **Protein**. My mom adds more protein to my portion prior to serving. She prepares extra meat ahead of time and portions it into freezer bags.
- **Calcium**. My mom uses finely ground egg shells for my calcium supplement. She adds phosphorus if necessary to maintain the correct balance between the two. These additives replace the bone meal you used to eat in dog food.
- **Omega 3 & Omega 6 Fatty Acids**. My mom adds additional fatty acids so I have a healthy skin and coat. She adds sardines, salmon, eggs, ground flax meal, and certain oils to my food.

Additives For Humans Only:

- Garlic & Onions
- Hot Peppers
- Salt (minimal) & Pepper

Your parents may need to add these to their food just prior to serving. All the recipes in the book do not include these ingredients or include them in minimal amounts. My mom adds other spices and flavor combinations to her recipes to make them flavorful without these ingredients.

Additives for Both of You.
Don't Forget to Pair Your Dining Experiences With One or More of the 4-Fs Throughout the Day:

- **Forward Moving.** Walk, jog, hike, bike, or swim together every day for at least 30-minutes.
- **Firmly Strengthened:** Create an all-around exercise program including at least 30 minutes of cardiovascular strengthening and muscle/joint strengthening at least 5 days per week. This is mostly for your parents, but you can join along.
- **Fully Flexible:** Spend 30 minutes everyday doing Yoga, stretching, or meditating together.
- **Fun Loving:** Play a structured fun and/or obedience game 2 or more times per day for at least 15 minutes.

When your mom gets to the recipe sections, she will see that each recipe specifies serving sizes based on the nutritional content and calorie amount to help her serve you the correct portion. The main meals add the "PLUS" items to achieve a more balanced experience.

Remember, no super-sizing allowed! After following the **4-PAWS-PLUS Plan** for a short time, you and your family will achieve Former-Couch-PAW-tato status.

My mom has just a few more basic guidelines next, and then you will be ready to get cooking and eating.

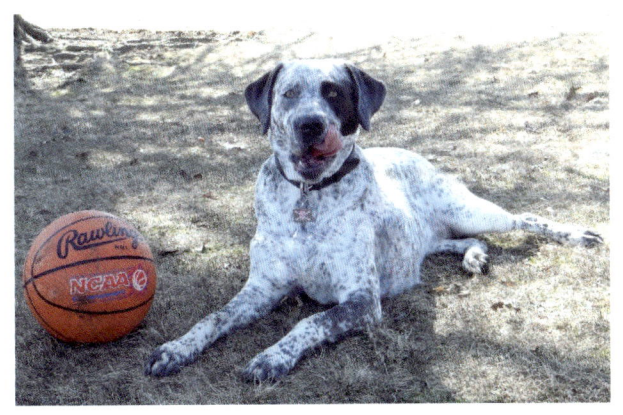

"I love to play basketball just like my mom used to in high school."

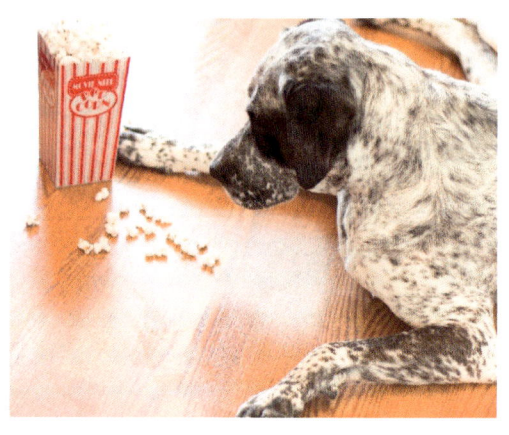

"It's Friday movie night with my favorite snack!"

4-PAWS-PLUS Plan™ Ten Basic Guidelines

"Here are ten basic guidelines my mom uses to keep me safe and well nourished."

You can learn more and find answers to all your questions by joining my mom's interactive online community at

www.eatyourowndogfood.net.

The community is a great way to share your dining experiences with other healthy-minded, dog enthusiasts who enjoy sharing great meals everyday with their best friend(s).

Ingredients

1. Use the freshest ingredients that fit into your budget.

My dad does all the grocery shopping for us. He purchases our meats and most staples at warehouse stores and local farmer's markets. Mom taught dad to read the labels for hidden sugar, salt, chemicals, "natural" flavorings, and preservatives found in cheaper store-brand foods. She made him return anything that contained this "goo," so now he carefully reads the label before purchasing.

2. Buy in bulk if you can afford it.

Online retailers offer bulk flours, meals, grains, and spices. My mom buys a lot and stores them in sealable plastic bags and airtight containers in the pantry and the freezer.

Preparation

3. Prepare, chop, and freeze ingredients so you always have them readily available.

My mom cooks beans, extra meat, spaghetti sauce, breads, muffins, crackers, rice, and pasta ahead of time and portions each in appropriately-sized containers for freezing. Dad chops many fresh herbs and spices, and vegetables, such as mushrooms, peppers, kale, and bok choy; she stores them in sealable bags in the freezer. Freezing makes the vegetables soggy when thawed so mom uses these only for soups, stews, and meals that do not require fresh raw ingredients.

4. Vary the four ingredient components you use in your meal preparation every day.

Mom uses different protein sources, grains, fruits, vegetables, and spices every day to create a new, pleasurable, and balanced experience. She knows how much I like her creation by how quickly I gobble it up and how clean I lick my bowl.

Additives

5. Create your own spice and vegetable mixes for your human portions.

Remember, dogs can't eat onions and garlic and hot peppers, which are favorites for many humans. Onion and garlic powder works well or sauté garlic and onions on the side or in a sauce to add to your human portion just before serving.

6. Ground egg shells are a great source of calcium for us.

Dogs need extra calcium for strong bones and teeth so save those egg shells. My mom cleans the shells, removes the inside membrane, microwaves the shells for about 20 seconds, and then lets them dry overnight. Dad grinds them to a fine powder using a spice/coffee grinder and stores the powder in an airtight container in the refrigerator. Mom removes the egg shell membrane because this creates a finer ground powder. She dries and crushes the membrane to add to my food a few times per week. One teaspoon of ground eggshells contains about 1,800 to 2,000 mg of calcium; she mixes the required amount in my food before serving.

Serving

7. We can't use eating utensils so be sure to chop our portions into bite-sized pieces.

Be sure to follow the portion size recommendations for each meal and adjust as necessary. Bite size depends on your size. I am a large dog, so I like big pieces and can devour a whole chicken breast without chopping; not recommended for my smaller friends who might need their food puréed!

8. We can't blow on our food to cool it off.

Before serving, my mom lets my food cool a bit until it is slightly warm to the touch to avoid injury. Be careful when microwaving food because it does not always heat evenly; there could be some hot spots….Ouch. Always wait until the food reaches the correct temperature throughout before serving.

Storage

9. Freeze portion-sized leftovers for quick meals later on.

My mom portions and freezes all of our leftovers for quick meals later in the week. I eat the same portion as my mom and dad so it is easy for us. If you are a smaller dog, your mom will have to make your portions smaller than their portions.

10. Snacks and Treats can be frozen in small batches.

Mom never runs out of treats for us to eat because she always makes extra and freezes them. We always have plenty on hand for snacking. Dad likes to snack a lot too.

Other Important PLUS Additives

These three additives are non-nutritional pluses to support your overall health. Be sure your parents perform these behaviors regularly and check with your veterinarian for his/her recommendations.

1. **Proper Oral Care.** My mom brushes my teeth every night to prevent tartar build up. Now that I eat real food, I don't get tartar, and I have the freshest breath ever. Mom has her own mix of toothpaste she developed that contains a little baking soda and peroxide. I also tug and play with flossy rope toys. Not sure if this helps other than stimulating my mouth and gums, but I sure love playing tug and chewing on them.

2. **Regular Health Checkups**. My parents take me to see my veterinarian regularly so I stay current on all my vaccinations and preventative treatments. Thankfully, my parents do not use topical flea and tick medication; no toxic chemicals here. They keep me clean and bathed, spray me with natural scents, and always check for ticks after playing outside.

3. **Regular Grooming.** I have an easy care coat so my parents don't need to take me to a groomer. My dad brushes my coat every week, and I get bathed 1-2 times per month with natural soaps and scents. My parents take me for lots of walks on many different surfaces so my nails stay filed down, slough, and grow naturally.

Now that you have the basics, it's time to get cooking.

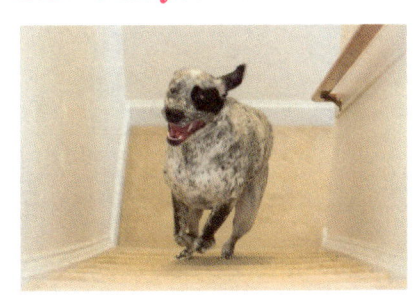

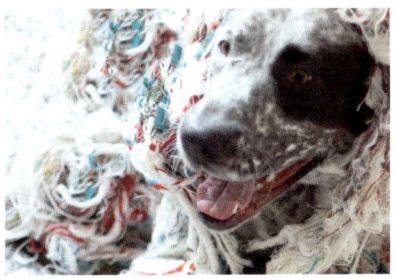

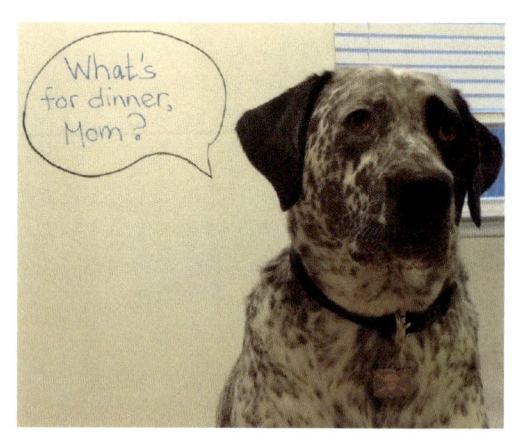

"These are some of my dinner favorites!"

Main ARF-Fair

Your mom can use these 20 recipes to create a main-dining experience for your family or use these as a first course for a complete dining event. Soups, stews, casseroles, and one-pot meals are a great way to pack in a lot of nutrition in a little bit of time.

Most of these meals satisfy all **4-PAWS**. Add the **PLUS** additives listed at the end of the recipe to make each one complete. The canine serving information and portion sizes for these main meals are based on **2 meals per day**.

If you have questions about any recipe contained in this book, please email your questions to us at **eatwithluna@gmail.com.**

Receive new main-meal recipes each week by joining our online community at
www.eatyourowndogfood.net

1. Garden Penne ARFredo with Chicken 44
2. BARKequed Chicken Pizza 46
3. Beef and VegeTAILble Spaghetti 48
4. Luna-Tuna Casserole 50
5. LenTAIL Pot Pie 52
6. Real Dogs Do Like Quiche 54
7. Hearty Beef SNOOP 56
8. Chicken-Vegetable BARK 58
9. Chicken PLAY-Cacciatore 60
10. Spicy Three-BELLY RUB Chili 62
11. Moroccan Chicken and Butternut Squash SNOOP 64
12. Brown Rice, Asparagus, and Goat Cheese Frittata 66
13. Pawed-Pork BARKeque 68
14. Sloppy Lunas 70
15. Turkey TAILmale Pie 72
16. Roast Pork with White Beans and Cranberries 74
17. MUTTball SNOOP with Greens 76
18. Fish and Corn CHOWDOWNner 78
19. GROWLED Buffalo Chicken Sliders 80
20. Faux-Ham, Sweet Potato, and Edamame Hash 82

Garden Penne ARFredo with Chicken

4-PAWS
This power-packed meal is high in protein, grains, and includes four great vegetables.

OVEN: N/A

EQUIPMENT: Large Skillet, Stockpot, Medium Saucepan

4 Skinless, Boneless Chicken Breast Halves
Salt and Pepper
Nonstick Cooking Spray
2 Medium Zucchini
2 Medium Yellow Squash
1 Red Bell Pepper
8 Thin Asparagus Spears

Sauce:
1 Tablespoon Olive Oil
2 Tablespoons Whole Grain Flour
1/2 Cup Homemade Chicken Broth
1 Cup Lowfat Milk
1 Cup Grated Parmesan Cheese
2 Tablespoons Lowfat Cream Cheese
2 Tablespoons Chopped Fresh Parsley
8 ounces of Brown Rice Penne Pasta

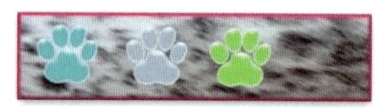

Heat a large skillet over medium heat. Coat skillet with cooking spray. Sprinkle chicken with salt and pepper. Add chicken and cook 4-5 minutes per side. Let stand 5 minutes then cut chicken across the grain into thin slices. Keep warm.

While the chicken is cooking, cook pasta according to package instructions. Drain and keep warm.

Cut squash in half lengthwise, core, cut in half, and then cut into thin strips. Cut bell pepper into thin strips, and remove ends of asparagus.

Heat a nonstick skillet or grill pan. Spray vegetables with olive oil, sprinkle with salt and pepper and saute'/grill for 2 minutes.

In the saucepan, combine the oil and flour. Using a whisk, gradually add broth until flour is dissolved, add milk, stir until thickens. Add both cheeses, stirring with a whisk until cheeses melt.

Toss with hot pasta, chicken and vegetables. Sprinkle with parsley, pepper, and a little more grated cheese.

SERVING SIZE:
Makes: 4 servings
Calories per serving: 500 cal

Human: 1 serving
Canine:
Extra Large: 1 serving
Large: 1 serving
Medium: 1/2 - 3/4 serving
Small: 1/4 - 1/2 serving

NUTRIENTS (per human serving):

Protein: 45 gm
Carbohydrate: 45 gm
Fat: 17 gm

Calcium: 426 mg
Phosphorus: 705 mg

SERVING SUGGESTIONS:
See the **Happy BARKday Bash** Theme-Day ARF-Fair (Page 133) .

PLUS Additives:

Canine:
Extra Large: 1 1/2 chicken breasts, 1 teaspoon of crushed egg shells

Large: 1 chicken breasts, 1 teaspoon crushed egg shells.

Medium: 1/2 - 3/4 chicken breast, 1/4 - 1/2 teaspoon crushed egg shells.

Small: 1/4-1/2 chicken breast, 1/8 - 1/4 teaspoon crushed egg shells.

Humans: Sprinkle with garlic powder

Pairing: Pair with Mixed Greens, Candied Walnut, and Pear Salad (Page 96) or a fruit salad.

Exercise: Be sure to add an after-dinner walk for 30 minutes.

LUNA SAYS:

"This is one of my favorite meals because I love, love, love cheese."

BARKequed Chicken Pizza

4-PAWS
Who knew pizza could be so good for you. The fresh ingredients including the crust and tangy chutney satisfy all **4-PAWS** with a punch of flavor.

OVEN: 400 Degrees F
EQUIPMENT: Bread Machine, Grater or Food Processor, Pizza Pan, Small Saucepan

1 Pizza Crust
3 Grilled Skinless, Boneless Chicken Breasts
2/3 Cup Roma Tomatoes, diced
1/3 Cup Mushrooms, chopped
3 ounces Shredded White Cheddar Cheese

Tomato-Pear Chutney:
2 Cups Roma Tomatoes
1 Pear, peeled, cored, diced
1/2 Cup Green Peppers, diced
3 Tablespoons Honey
3 Tablespoons Cider Vinegar
1/8 teaspoon Jamaican Jerk Seasoning

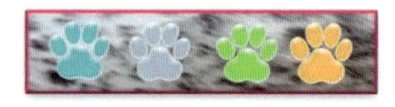

Prework: **Make a 12-inch whole wheat pizza shell using the recipe included with your bread machine.** Prebake the shell for 7-8 minutes prior to using.

Sprinkle the chicken breasts with salt and pepper. Spray a skillet or grill pan with cooking spray. Cook chicken 4-5 minutes per side until done. Let cool. When cooled, shred with two forks.

Prepare the tomato chutney. Dice the 2 roma tomatoes and place in the small sauce pan. Add honey, cider vinegar, and Jerk seasoning. Bring to a boil and reduce heat to medium. Cook 20 minutes until thickened.

Preheat the oven. Place the prebaked crust on pizza pan. Spread with chutney, top with chicken, diced tomatoes, and grated cheese. Bake for 10-12 minutes until cheese melts.

SERVING SIZE:
Makes: 8 slices
Calories per slice: 280

Human: 2 slices
Canine:
Extra Large: 2 1/2 slices
Large: 2 slices
Medium: 1 slice
Small: 1/2 slice

NUTRIENTS (per human serving):

Protein: 10 gm
Carbohydrate: 26 gm
Fat: 10 gm

Calcium: 98 mg
Phosphorus: 348 mg

SERVING SUGGESTIONS:
Pair with a green salad or fruit salad.

TIPS:
Using your bread machine, make ahead and freeze a batch of pizza shells. Prebake the shells in a 400 Degrees F oven for 8 min. Cool completely and wrap in plastic.

Experiment with other homemade pizza sauces and toppings.

PLUS Additives:

Canine:
Extra Large: 2 chicken breasts, 1 teaspoon of crushed egg shells

Large: 1 1/2 chicken breasts, 1 teaspoon crushed egg shells.

Medium:
1 chicken breast, 1/4 - 1/2 teaspoon crushed egg shells.

Small: 1/4-1/2 chicken breast, 1/8 - 1/4 teaspoon crushed egg shells.

Humans: Sprinkle with garlic and onion powder and red pepper flakes for an extra spicy experience.

Exercise: Play a game of hide and seek with a favorite toy.

LUNA SAYS:

"I'm glad my mom loves pizza. We have a different type of pizza once a week. I don't have hands, so she cuts my slices into smaller, bite-sized pieces."

Beef and VegeTAILble Spaghetti

4-PAWS
This versatile sauce is packed with vegetables, beef, and a ton of spices. This one deserves a 4-PAW rating, a no-brainer here.

OVEN: N/A
EQUIPMENT: Large Saucepan, Large Stockpot

1 pound Ground Beef
2 Cups Carrots, grated
1 Cup Mushrooms, chopped
1 Each: Red, Yellow, and Green
  Pepper, chopped
2 Roma Tomatoes, chopped
4 6-ounce cans Tomato Paste
  (no salt or sugar added)
1 Cup Pear or Apple Purée
2 Teaspoons Dried Basil
2 teaspoons Dried Oregano
2 teaspoons Italian Seasoning
2 teaspoons Dried Parsley
1 teaspoon Ground Pepper
1 package Brown Rice
  Spaghetti
Grated Parmesan or Pecorino-Romano Cheese

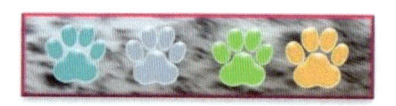

In the large sauce pan, brown ground beef and drain off fat. Add carrots, mushrooms, peppers, and tomatoes. Saute' with the beef for 5 minutes.

Stir in tomato paste and 8 cans of water. Add more water if needed if the sauce is too thick

Add fruit purée and spices. Heat to boiling, reduce heat, partially cover and simmer for 40 minutes.

In the large stockpot, cook spaghetti according to package directions.

Serve with a little grated parmesan cheese.

NOTE: This recipe makes a large pot of sauce. See tips section for other uses and what to do with leftovers.

SERVING SIZE:
Serving Size: 1 1/2 cups of Sauce and 1 cup pasta
Calories per serving: 320

Human: 1 serving
Canine:
Extra Large: 1 serving
Large: 1 serving
Medium: 1/2 - 3/4 serving
Small: 1/4 - 1/2 serving

NUTRIENTS (per human serving):

Protein: 15 gm
Carbohydrate: 48 gm
Fat: 8 gm

Calcium: 45 mg
Phosphorus: 281 mg

SERVING SUGGESTIONS:
See the **ItailWAGGIN' Feast** Theme Day ARF-Fair (Page 133).

TIPS:
This sauce can be used for a baked lasagna or even pizza.

Freeze the extra in a larger container for use in other meals or make small individual serving leftover portions for quick meals.

PLUS Additives:

Canine:
Extra Large: 2/3 pound ground beef, 1 teaspoon of crushed egg shells

Large: 1/2 pound ground beef, 1 teaspoon crushed egg shells.

Medium: 1/4 ground beef, 1/4 - 1/2 teaspoon crushed egg shells.

Small: 1/8 pound ground beef, 1/8 - 1/4 teaspoon crushed egg shells.

Humans: Sprinkle with garlic and onion powder and red pepper flakes for an extra spicy experience.

Exercise: Play a good game of tug with a rope toy or old rag.

LUNA SAYS:

"I never turn down mom's spaghetti sauce. It's a triple-bowl-licking meal."

Eat Your Own Dog Food Series

Luna-Tuna Casserole

4-PAWS
We don't use many canned items. This spin on the classic tuna casserole takes the comfort and nutritional value up a few notches.

OVEN: 350 Degrees F
EQUIPMENT: Electric Pressure Cooker, Large Skillet, Large Bowl, 13 x 9 Baking Dish

1 Tablespoon Olive Oil
1 Red Pepper, diced
1 Green Pepper, diced
3 Cups Mushrooms, chopped
3 Roma Tomatoes, diced
2 Tablespoons Dried Marjoram
1/4 Cup Dried Cilantro
2 Cups Cooked Black-Eyed Peas
4 Cans Tuna, drained
10-ounces of Brown Rice Pasta Shells, cooked
4 Cups of Milk
1 Cup Apple Purée
4 Tablespoons Hard White Wheat Flour
Nonstick Cooking Spray

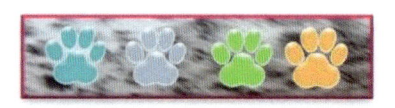

1 Cup Almonds, grated
1/2 Cup Pecorino-Romano Cheese, grated

Cook black-eyed peas ahead of time in the electric pressure cooker and cook pasta according to package directions.

Heat oil in the large skillet. Sauté diced peppers, mushrooms, and tomatoes for 5 minutes. Add marjoram and cilantro.

Add milk to the vegetable mix. In a small cup, dissolve flour in 1/2 cup of water. Pour into milk and vegetable mixture. Heat thoroughly and cook until the mixture thickens.

In the large bowl, toss cooked pasta, tuna, black-eyed peas. Mix in the milk and vegetable mixture. When thoroughly mixed. Pour into prepared baking dish.

Top with grated almonds and sprinkle with Pecorino-Romano cheese.

Bake for 45 minutes or until cooked through.

SERVING SIZE:
Makes: 12 servings
Calories per serving: 375

Human: 1 serving
Canine:
Extra Large: 1 serving
Large: 1 serving
Medium: 1/2 - 3/4 serving
Small: 1/4 - 1/2 serving

NUTRIENTS
(per human serving):

Protein: 23 gm
Carbohydrate: 48 gm
Fat: 11 gm

Calcium: 193 mg
Phosphorus: 434 mg

TIP:
For any of the dishes that contain beans or peas cook them in your pressure cooker before hand and freeze cooled, cooked beans and peas in recipe-sized containers. Just thaw and use.

PLUS Additives:

Canine:
Extra Large: 1 1/2 cans of tuna, 1 teaspoon of crushed egg shells

Large: 1 can tuna, 1 teaspoon crushed egg shells.

Medium: 3/4 can tuna, 1/4 - 1/2 teaspoon crushed egg shells.

Small: 1/4 - 1/2 can of tuna, 1/8 - 1/4 teaspoon crushed egg shells.

Humans: Sprinkle with garlic and onion powder.

Exercise: Go for a nature hike for about 30-minutes.

LUNA SAYS:

"This casserole gives me a ton of energy, be ready to play or go for a long run or walk. You might want to save this meal for the weekend when we have more time to expend our energy."

LenTAIL Pot Pie

4-PAWS
This vegetarian dish will fool even the most devoted carnivore. The lentils provide a great source of low-fat protein and are high in complex carbohydrates.

OVEN: 375 Degrees F
EQUIPMENT: Electric Pressure Cooker, Medium Stockpot, Medium Microwave Safe Container with Cover, Large Skillet, Electric Mixer or Stick Blender, 13 x 9 Baking Pan or 2-Quart Casserole

1 1/2 pounds of Sweet Potatoes
2/3 Cup Lowfat Milk
1/2 teaspoon Salt
2 Cups Cooked Green Lentils
1 Tablespoon Olive Oil
1/2 Cup Celery, chopped
2 Cups Mushrooms, chopped
4 Cups Frozen Mixed Vegetables
1 1/2 Cups Vegetable Broth or Water (divided)
1 Cup Pear Purée
3 Tablespoons Whole Wheat Flour
2 Tablespoons Dry Sherry

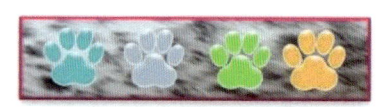

1 Tablespoon Soy Sauce
1 Tablespoon Tomato Paste
1 teaspoon dried chopped Thyme

Prepare lentils ahead of time using the electric pressure cooker and microwave mixed vegetables. Prepare pear purée. Set both aside.

Peel and cube potatoes. Place in water and boil for 20 minutes or until very tender. Drain, return to pan, and add milk and salt. Mash potatoes with an electric mixer of stick blender. Set aside.

Filling:
Heat oil in the large skillet. Add celery and mushrooms. Cook for 7 minutes. stirring occasionally.

Stir in cooked mixed vegetables, 1 cup of water (or broth), pear purée, sherry, soy sauce, tomato paste, thyme, and cooked lentils. In a small cup, mix flour with 1/2 cup water (broth). Stir in flour mixture and cook until it thickens. Spoon lentil mixture into baking pan or casserole. Top with sweet potato mixture spreading evenly.

Bake for 25 minutes until warmed through and bubbly.

SERVING SIZE:
Makes: 6 servings
Calories per serving: 300

Human: 1 serving
Canine:
Extra Large: 1 serving
Large: 1 serving
Medium: 1/2 - 3/4 serving
Small: 1/4 - 1/2 serving

NUTRIENTS
(per human serving):

Protein: 11 gm
Carbohydrate: 57 gm
Fat: 3 gm

Calcium: 103 mg
Phosphorus: 278 mg

SERVING SUGGESTIONS:
See the **Grande Blue Gascon Plate Special** Theme-Day ARF-Fair (Page 133).

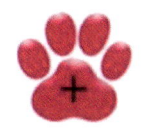

PLUS Additives:

Canine:
Extra Large: 2 cans of sardines, 1 teaspoon of crushed egg shells

Large: 1 1/2 cans sardines, 1 teaspoon crushed egg shells.

Medium: 1 can of sardines, 1/4 - 1/2 teaspoon crushed egg shells.

Small: 1/4 - 1/2 can of sardines, 1/8 - 1/4 teaspoon crushed egg shells.

Humans: Sprinkle with garlic and onion powder.

Exercise: Try some Dog Yoga.

LUNA SAYS:

"We like vegetarian meals too; however, mom always adds meat to mine before serving, so I'm only half vegetarian."

Real-Dogs-Do-Like Quiche

4-PAWS
Again, a great vegetarian meal that is packed full of protein and vegetables. Using lowfat milk will lower the fat a bit.

OVEN: 400 Degrees F
EQUIPMENT: Large Skillet, Medium Bowl, 9-inch Pie Pan or Tart Pan

Crust:
See crust instructions for Pear and Apple Galette with Olive Oil Crust (Page 124).

Filling:
- 2 Tablespoons Olive Oil
- 1 Medium Zucchini
- 1 Yellow Squash
- 1/2 Cup Mushrooms
- 1 Cup Frozen Shelled Edamame, thawed
- 3 Large Eggs
- 1 1/2 Cups of Milk
- 1 Tablespoon Hard White Wheat Flour
- 1 Cup Pecorino-Romano Cheese, grated

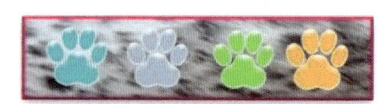

Prepare crust and line the 9-inch pie or tart pan.

Shred squash and finely chop the mushrooms. In the large skillet, heat oil over medium-high heat. Sauté the vegetables for about 4 minutes.

Add edamame, cook and stir until combined, about 1 minute. Season with a little salt and pepper. Let mixture cool.

In the medium bowl, whisk eggs, milk, and flour until smooth. Stir in vegetable mixture and 3/4 cup of the cheese. Pour into crust and sprinkle with remaining 1/4 cup of cheese.

Bake for 50 minutes until puffy and pale golden brown. Tent with foil for the last 15 minutes of baking if necessary to prevent over browning.

Let cool at least 30 minutes before serving.

Eat Your Own Dog Food Series

SERVING SIZE:
Makes: 6 servings
Calories per serving: 370

Human: 1 serving
Canine:
Extra Large: 1 serving
Large: 1 serving
Medium: 1/2 - 3/4 serving
Small: 1/4 - 1/2 serving

NUTRIENTS (per human serving):

Protein: 16 gm
Carbohydrate: 23 gm
Fat: 24 gm

Calcium: 290 mg
Phosphorus: 367 mg

SERVING SUGGESTIONS:
Serve with a mixed green salad.

TIPS:
Use the same egg and milk base, but vary your vegetables and fruit purée, and cheese to make your own unique combinations.

PLUS Additives:

Canine:
Extra Large: 1 1/2 chicken breasts, 1 teaspoon of crushed egg shells

Large: 1 chicken breast, 1 teaspoon crushed egg shells.

Medium: 1/2 - 3/4 chicken breast, 1/4 - 1/2 teaspoon crushed egg shells.

Small: 1/4 - 1/2 chicken breast, 1/8 - 1/4 teaspoon crushed egg shells.

Humans: Sprinkle with garlic and onion powder.

Exercise: Play the shell game by hiding a favorite toy or treat under three plastic containers.

LUNA SAYS:

"I'm a real dog, and I really do love my quiche with mom's crispy crust with a side of meat, of course."

Hearty Beef SNOOP

4-PAWS
Definitely a 4-PAW pleaser. The added beans and peas up the nutritional value and flavor too.

OVEN: N/A
EQUIPMENT: Large Stockpot

2 pounds of Stew Beef, cooked
8 Cups of Water/Broth
1 Cups Lima Beans, cooked
1 Cups Field Peas, cooked
4 Medium Carrots, sliced
1 Cup Frozen Green Peas
1 Cup Frozen Corn
1 Large Sweet Potato, peeled and diced
1/2 Cup Green Pepper, diced
2 Roma Tomatoes, chopped
1 6-ounce Can Tomato Paste
1 Cup Apple Puree
1/2 teaspoon Ground Black Pepper
2 teaspoons Marjoram

3 teaspoons Arrowroot Starch
Water

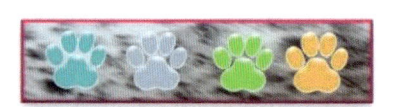

_____

Precook lima beans and field peas in electric pressure cooker according to instructions.

Precook beef in electric pressure cooker. Add beef, 1-inch of water, salt, and pepper to pressure cooker and cook on Beef setting.

Place water/broth through spices into a large stock pot. Use a combination of water and strained broth (fat removed) from cooking your beef in the pressure cooker.

Bring to boil and simmer for 25 minutes until carrots and potatoes are cooked. Add beef and more water if needed have enough broth and simmer for 5 more minutes.

Optional: For a thicker stew-like texture, in a small cup, mix 3 teaspoons arrowroot starch with enough water to dissolve. Stir into pot and simmer a few minutes until thickened.

SERVING SIZE:
Makes: 8 (1 1/2 cup) servings
Calories per serving: 405

Human: 1 serving
Canine:
Extra Large: 1 serving
Large: 1 serving
Medium: 1/2 - 3/4 serving
Small: 1/4 - 1/2 serving

NUTRIENTS
(per human serving):

Protein: 34 gm
Carbohydrate: 52 gm
Fat: 7 gm

Calcium: 92 mg
Phosphorus: 450 mg

SERVING SUGGESTIONS:
This is great on its own.

TIPS:
Precooking and freezing the beef, lima beans and field peas ahead of time saves considerable cooking time.

Freeze in small portion size containers or resealable storage bags.

PLUS Additives:

Canine:
Extra Large: 5 ounces of beef, 1 teaspoon of crushed egg shells

Large: 4 ounces of beef, 1 teaspoon crushed egg shells.

Medium: 3 ounces of beef, 1/4 - 1/2 teaspoon crushed egg shells.

Small: 1 - 2 ounces of beef, 1/8 - 1/4 teaspoon crushed egg shells.

Humans: Sprinkle with garlic and onion powder.

Exercise: Take a jog around the park and stop off at the dog park for 15 minutes.

LUNA SAYS:

"I like to eat this after a long walk on a cold day."

Chicken-Vegetable BARK

4-PAWS
There are plenty of vegetables and flavor in this baked casserole so we don't really miss the fruit. The spices and coconut truly comfort and satisfy

OVEN: 375 Degrees F
EQUIPMENT: Large Nonstick Skillet, Medium Stock Pot, Large Bowl, 13 x 9 Baking Dish

10 ounces Brown Rice Pasta Springs, cooked
6 Boneless, Skinless Chicken Breasts, cooked and shredded
1 Tablespoon Olive Oil
3 Cups Butternut Squash, peeled and cubed
1 Cup Shredded Parsnips
4 Cups Kale, rinsed and chopped
1 teaspoon Dried Rubbed Sage
1 teaspoon Dried Parsley
1/8 teaspoon Cinnamon
Pinch of Cloves
Pinch of Nutmeg
1/2 teaspoon Black Pepper
Nonstick Cooking Spray

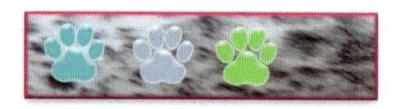

Sauce:
2 Tablespoons Olive Oil
4 Tablespoons Hard White Wheat Flour
1 Cup Homemade Broth
2 Cups Milk
2 Cups Cottage Cheese

Topping:
1/4 Cup Grated Pecorino Romano Cheese
1 Cup Almonds, grated
1/4 Cup Unsweetened Coconut, shredded

Precook chicken in electric pressure cooker and precook pasta the medium stock pot per package direction. Set aside.

Heat olive oil in the large skilled. Sauté all vegetables for 5-10 minutes. Stir in spices.

Place cooked chicken, cooked pasta, and vegetable mixture in the large bowl.

To make sauce, in the medium sauce pan, heat olive oil.

Mix in flour and then whisk in milk until smooth. Cook until heated through. Stir in cottage cheese. Pour into large bowl, combine thoroughly and pour into the baking dish prepared with cooking spray. Sprinkle with grated cheese, almonds, and coconut.

Bake 30-35 minutes until browned.

SERVING SIZE:
Makes: 12 servings
Calories per serving: 432

Human: 1 serving
Canine:
Extra Large: 1 serving
Large: 1 serving
Medium: 1/2 - 3/4 serving
Small: 1/4 - 1/2 serving

NUTRIENTS (per human serving):

Protein: 26 gm
Carbohydrate: 44 gm
Fat: 18 gm

Calcium: 187 mg
Phosphorus: 403 mg

SERVING SUGGESTIONS:
This stands alone. Savor the unique combination of flavors.

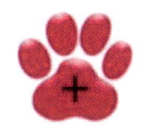

PLUS Additives:

Canine:
Extra Large: 1 1/2 chicken breasts, 1 teaspoon of crushed egg shells

Large: 1 chicken breasts, 1 teaspoon crushed egg shells.

Medium: 3/4 chicken breast, 1/4 - 1/2 teaspoon crushed egg shells.

Small: 1/4-1/2 chicken breast, 1/8 - 1/4 teaspoon crushed egg shells.

Humans: Sprinkle with garlic and onion powder.

Exercise: Don't forget your after dinner walk and fetch in the yard.

LUNA SAYS:

"I love this creamy stick-to-my-ribs meal. It's hard to eat just one serving. "

Chicken PLAY-Cacciatore

4-PAWS
This is a great one-pot meal that is a snap to make in an electric pressure cooker. No more slow cooking here.

OVEN: N/A
EQUIPMENT: 8-Quart Electric Pressure Cooker, Large Skillet

8 Chicken Thighs, bone-in, skinned
8 Chicken Drumsticks, skinned
Salt and Pepper
1 Tablespoon olive oil
Nonstick Cooking Spray
8-ounce package of Mushrooms, quartered
1 Green Pepper, vertically sliced
1 Red Pepper, vertically sliced
Sauce:
1/2 dry cooking wine
4 Roma Tomatoes, chopped
1 Cup Water or Broth
1 Cup Apple Purée
1/3 Cup Hard White Wheat Flour
1 teaspoon Dried Oregano
1 teaspoon Dried Chopped Thyme
4 Cups Cooked Brown Rice

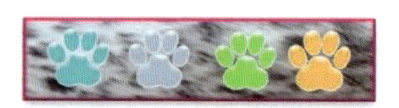

Heat olive oil in the large skillet. Sprinkle chicken with salt and pepper. Brown chicken about 5 minutes until slightly brown.

Place chicken in electric pressure cooker coated with cooking spray. Top with mushrooms.

In the same saucepan, sauté peppers for 5 minutes. Add wine, cook for 1-2 minutes. Stir in water/broth, tomatoes, flour, and spices.

Pour over chicken and mushrooms. Cook in pressure cooker for 20 minutes. Let pressure release on own (about 30 minutes). Serve with pasta.

Eat Your Own Dog Food Series

SERVING SIZE:
Makes: 8 servings plus 1/2 cup of pasta
Calories per serving: 542

Human: 1 serving
Canine:
Extra Large: 1 serving
Large: 1 serving
Medium: 1/2 serving
Small: 1/4 serving

NUTRIENTS
(per human serving):

Protein: 60 gm
Carbohydrate: 42 gm
Fat: 15 gm

Calcium: 47 mg
Phosphorus: 630 mg

SERVING SUGGESTIONS:
Cut portion to 1 piece of chicken and 1/4 cup rice for lower protein and calories. Serve with a mixed green salad.

TIPS:
Be sure to remove the bones for your best friend before serving. Leave the cartilage for added nutritional value.

PLUS Additives:

Canine:
Extra Large: 1 chicken thigh, 1 teaspoon of crushed egg shells

Large: 1/2 - 3/4 chicken thigh, 1 teaspoon crushed egg shells.

Medium: 1/2 - 1/4 chicken thigh, 1/4 - 1/2 teaspoon crushed egg shells.

Small: 1/8-1/4 chicken thigh, 1/8 - 1/4 teaspoon crushed egg shells.

Humans: Sprinkle with garlic and onion powder.

Exercise: Consistent with the recipe name, a game of tag would be in order. Clear out a space to run and jump around.

LUNA SAYS:

"The tomato base is my favorite and coats my bowl for some extra licking."

Main ARF-Fair

Eat Your Own Dog Food Series

Spicy Three-BELLY RUB Chili

4-PAWS
With three types of beans and meat, this chili is sure to provide the extra energy to get you through the day. It's a definite 4-PAW pleaser

OVEN: N/A

EQUIPMENT: Medium Skillet, Large Stockpot

1 pound Ground Beef
1 Cup each of Green, Red, and Yellow Peppers, diced
1 Tablespoon Jalapeno Pepper, diced
4 1/2 Cups Water
1 1/2 Cups Homemade Chicken Broth
1 6-ounce Can Tomato Paste
2 Tablespoons Lime Juice
2 Tablespoons Agave Nectar
1 Cup Blueberry Purée
2 Tablespoons Ground Cumin
2 1/2 Tablespoons Chilli Powder
4 teaspoons Paprika
4 teaspoons Dried Basil
2 teaspoons Dried Cilantro
1/2 teaspoon Ground Oregano

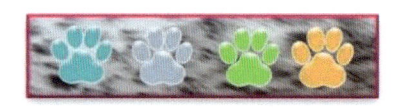

2 Cups each of Pinto, Black, and Kidney Beans, cooked

Prepare beans in electric pressure cooker ahead of time.

In the large skillet, cook ground beef until done and drain fat.

In the large stock pot, heat oil and sauté peppers until tender. Add water, broth, tomato paste, lime juice, agave nectar, fruit purée, and seasonings.

Add cooked ground beef and beans. Simmer for 30 minutes. For thicker chilli, mix 3 Tablespoons of arrowroot starch with enough water to dissolve. Stir into chili. Cook a few minutes more until thickened.

SERVING SIZE:
Makes: 12 (1/12 cup) servings
Calories per serving: 435

Human: 1 serving
Canine:
Extra Large: 1 serving
Large: 1 serving
Medium: 1/2 - 3/4 serving
Small: 1/4 - 1/2 serving

NUTRIENTS (per human serving):

Protein: 28 gm
Carbohydrate: 63 gm
Fat: 7 gm

Calcium: 114 mg
Phosphorus: 451 mg

SERVING SUGGESTIONS:
Serve with a sprinkle of cheddar cheese.

TIPS:
Make all of your beans ahead of time using an electric pressure cooker. Freeze recipe-sized portions so you always have some on hand. For this recipe, no need to thaw, just dump them in the pot.

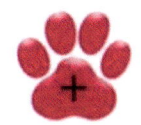

PLUS Additives:

Canine:
Extra Large: 6 ounces of beef, 1 teaspoon of crushed egg shells

Large: 5 ounces of beef, 1 teaspoon crushed egg shells.

Medium: 4 ounces of beef, 1/4 - 1/2 teaspoon crushed egg shells.

Small: 2-3 ounces of beef, 1/8 - 1/4 teaspoon crushed egg shells.

Humans: Sprinkle with garlic and onion powder.

Exercise: After the belly rubs, put on your favorite music and have a dance party.

LUNA SAYS:

"Mom's chili rocks, especially the extra belly rubs that go along with it."

Moroccan Chicken and Butternut Squash SNOOP

4-PAWS
A great spicy one-pot meal ready in no time. The dark chicken meat amps up the phosphorus.

OVEN: N/A
EQUIPMENT: Large Stockpot

2 Tablespoon Olive Oil
8 Skinless, Boneless Chicken Thighs, cut into bite-sized pieces
1 teaspoon Ground Cumin
1/8 teaspoon Cinnamon
1 teaspoon Ground Pepper
3 Cups Butternut Squash, peeled and cubed (1/2 inch)
1 Zucchini, diced
2 Cups Bok Choy, chopped
1 Cup Mushrooms, chopped
8 Cups Water
4 Tablespoons Tomato Paste
2/3 Cup Quinoa, rinsed
2 teaspoons Dried Basil
1/2 teaspoon Salt
2 teaspoons Grated Orange Rind

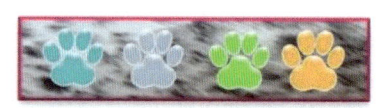

In a large stock pot, heat oil. Add chicken and cook for 4-5 minutes until done. Add cumin, cinnamon, and pepper. Cook 1-2 minutes.

Add squash, zucchini, bok choy, and mushrooms. Stir until heated.

Add water, tomato paste, quinoa, basil, salt, and orange rind.

Simmer for 20 minutes until quinoa and squash are cooked.

SERVING SIZE:
Makes: 6 (2 cup) servings
Calories per serving: 350

Human: 1 serving
Canine:
Extra Large: 1 serving
Large: 1 serving
Medium: 1/2 serving
Small: 1/4 serving

NUTRIENTS (per human serving):

Protein: 41 gm
Carbohydrate: 21 gm
Fat: 13 gm

Calcium: 97 mg
Phosphorus: 466 mg

SERVING SUGGESTIONS:
Serve with half a toasted flatbread PAW-ket (Page 112).

TIPS:
Vary the meat and vegetables to change it up. For a vegan meal, try diced tofu or seitan.

PLUS Additives:

Canine:
Extra Large: 2 chicken thighs, 1 teaspoon of crushed egg shells

Large: 1 1/2 chicken thighs, 1 teaspoon crushed egg shells.

Medium: 1 chicken thigh, 1/4 - 1/2 teaspoon crushed egg shells.

Small: 1/4-1/2 chicken thigh, 1/8 - 1/4 teaspoon crushed egg shells.

Humans: Sprinkle with garlic and onion powder.

Exercise: Learn a new trick, both of you!

LUNA SAYS:

"I can smell mom cooking this meal a mile away. The spicier the better."

Main ARF-Fair

Brown Rice, Asparagus, and Goat Cheese Frittata

4-PAWS

Great for breakfast or brunch; the richness of the goat cheese changes it up a bit and makes this one a favorite.

OVEN: 325 Degrees F
EQUIPMENT: Medium Bowl, Whisk, Large Nonstick Skillet (oven safe)

2 Tablespoons Water
1/2 teaspoon Salt
1/4 teaspoon Ground Black Pepper
6 Large Eggs

Nonstick Cooking Spray
1 Cup Asparagus, sliced (1/2 inch)
1/2 Cup Mushrooms, chopped
1 Roma Tomato, chopped
2 Cups Fresh Spinach
1 Cup Cooked Brown Rice
1 teaspoon Lemon Rind
1 teaspoon Dried Basil
1/4 Cup Crumbled Goat Cheese (1-2 ounces)

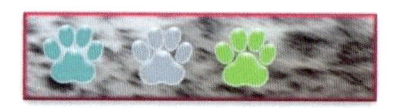

In the medium bowl, whisk the water, salt, pepper, and eggs. Set aside.

Heat the large skillet over medium heat. Spray with cooking spray.

Sauté asparagus and mushrooms for 3 minutes. Add the tomatoes, spinach, rice, basil, and lemon rind. Cook until heated through.

Reduce heat and pat vegetable mixture into an even layer in the pan.

Sprinkle with goat cheese and pour egg mixture on top. Cover and continue to cook over medium heat about 4 minutes until almost set.

Remove cover. Wrap handle of pan with foil and place in the oven under a preheated broiler. Broil for about 4 minutes until brown and set.

SERVING SIZE:
Makes: 4 servings
Calories per serving: 250

Human: 1 serving
Canine:
Extra Large: 1 serving
Large: 1 serving
Medium: 1/2 serving
Small: 1/4 serving

NUTRIENTS (per human serving):

Protein: 18 gm
Carbohydrate: 18 gm
Fat: 13 gm

Calcium: 200 mg
Phosphorus: 309 mg

SERVING SUGGESTIONS:
Add some fresh berries to finish this one off.

TIPS:
Vary the vegetables and cheese you use for this one. Try some quinoa instead of the rice.

If you are a true carnivore, add some chicken or Faux-sausage.

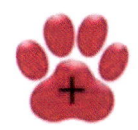

PLUS Additives:

Canine:
Extra Large: 2 cans of sardines, 1 teaspoon of crushed egg shells

Large: 1 1/2 cans sardines, 1 teaspoon crushed egg shells.

Medium: 1 can of sardines, 1/4 - 1/2 teaspoon crushed egg shells.

Small: 1/4-1/2 can of sardines, 1/8 - 1/4 teaspoon crushed egg shells.

Humans: Sprinkle with garlic and onion powder.

Exercise: Try a little homemade agility exercise in your backyard.

LUNA SAYS:

"My mom always pairs sardines with my eggs, well, actually dad adds the sardines."

Pawed-Pork BARKeque

4-PAWS
The homemade sauce and lean pork sirloin make this a low-fat and low-sodium favorite that won't last long.

OVEN: N/A
EQUIPMENT: Electric Pressure Cooker, Large Skillet

2 1/2 pound Pork Sirloin Tip Roast
1 Tablespoon Paprika
2 teaspoons Dry Mustard
Sprinkle of Salt and Pepper

Sauce:
1 Cup Water
3 Tablespoons Cider Vinegar
1/2 Cup Brown or Yellow Mustard
1/4 Cup Tomato Paste
3 Tablespoons Honey
1/2 teaspoon Salt
1/4 teaspoon Ground Pepper

Season the pork roast, add a little water and cook in electric pressure cooker. Roast should easily pull apart.

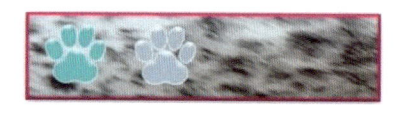

While the pork is cooking, make the sauce.

In a large skillet, combine all sauce ingredients. Simmer gently for about 10 minutes. Remove from heat.

Shred the pork roast using two forks. Add pork to the sauce mixture and stir until coated.

Serve in a Flatbread PAW-ket (Page 112) or with Almond-Wheat ROLLovers (Page 111).

SERVING SIZE:
Makes: 6 servings
Calories per serving: 265
With 1 Almond ROLLover: 385

Human: 1 serving
Canine:
Extra Large: 2 servings
Large: 1 1/2 servings
Medium: 1 serving
Small: 1/2 - 3/4 serving

NUTRIENTS
(per human serving):

Protein: 48 gm
Carbohydrate: 33 gm
Fat: 9 gm

Calcium: 26 mg
Phosphorus: 469 mg

SERVING SUGGESTIONS:
See the **Backyard BARKeque** Theme-Day ARF-Fair (Page 133) to make this a 4 PAW meal.

TIPS:
Add one of the VegeTAILble sides to make this a complete meal. This goes well with the drunken green beans. Use the skimmed pork broth to cook the beans.

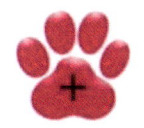

PLUS Additives:

Canine:
Extra Large: 1 teaspoon of crushed egg shells

Large: 1 teaspoon crushed egg shells.

Medium: 1/4 - 1/2 teaspoon crushed egg shells.

Small: 1/8 - 1/4 teaspoon crushed egg shells.

Humans: Sprinkle with garlic and onion powder.

Exercise: Time for a 30-minute interval walk. Alternate walking for 5-minutes and jogging for 5-minutes. For low impact, alternate power walking with walking.

LUNA SAYS:

"Mom's barbeque is the best. It's a definite return-to-lick-the-bowl experience. I would lick my fingers too if I had them."

Sloppy Lunas

4-PAWS

A great alternative to plain old sloppy joes. Crank it up a notch by adding cooked lentils and a minty sauce. Try ground lamb next time.

OVEN: N/A
EQUIPMENT: Electric Pressure Cooker, Large Skillet

2 Cups Lentils, cooked
1/2 Cup Green Pepper, finely diced
1/2 Cup Red Pepper, finely diced
1/4 teaspoon Salt
1/4 teaspoon Ground Black Pepper
1/2 pound Lean Ground Beef or Ground Lamb
1 teaspoon Dried Cumin
1 teaspoon Dried Thyme
4 Roma Tomatoes, diced
1/2 Cup Water

Sauce:
1/2 Cup Plain Nonfat Yogurt
1 Cup Cucumbers, thinly diced
Pinch of Dried Mint (optional)

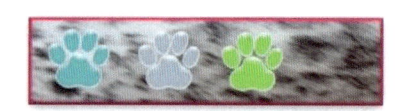

Precook lentils in the electric pressure cooker. Set aside.

Prepare sauce by mixing all ingredients together. Chill until ready to serve.

Heat the large skillet over medium heat and cook the meat until done. Drain fat. Add peppers, salt, and pepper. Sauté for 5 minutes longer.

Add tomatoes water, cumin, and thyme. Cook for 5 minutes. Add cooked lentils and cook 10 more minutes until thick.

Serve with Flatbread PAW-kets (Page 112). Spoon 1 Tablespoon of sauce in each half and fill with meat and lentil mixture.

SERVING SIZE:

Makes: 4 servings
Calories per serving: 280
With 1 Flatbread PAW-ket: 467

Human: 1 serving
Canine: 1 serving
Extra Large: 1 serving
Large: 1 serving
Medium: 1/2 serving
Small: 1/4 - 1/8 serving

NUTRIENTS
(per human serving):

Protein: 23 gm
Carbohydrate: 28 gm
Fat: 9 gm

Calcium: 41 mg
Phosphorus: 308 mg

SERVING SUGGESTIONS:

Serve with a small apple, pear, and dried fig fruit salad sprinkled with cinnamon.

TIPS:

This meal needs additional ground meat added to boost the protein for canines. Cook an extra pound of meat ahead of time and freeze in serving-size resealable bags.

PLUS Additives:

Canine:
Extra Large: 6 ounces of beef, 1 teaspoon of crushed egg shells

Large: 5 ounces of beef, 1 teaspoon crushed egg shells.

Medium: 4 ounces of beef, 1/4 - 1/2 teaspoon crushed egg shells.

Small: 2-3 ounces of beef, 1/8 - 1/4 teaspoon crushed egg shells.

Humans: Sprinkle with garlic and onion powder.

Exercise: Time for a 30-minute nature walk to uncover some new smells.

LUNA SAYS:

"Add beef to anything and it will taste great."

Turkey TAIL-male Pie

4-PAWS
A southwest favorite packed with beans and vegetables. Enjoy the cornmeal topping.

OVEN: 425 Degrees F
EQUIPMENT: Electric Pressure Cooker, Large Skillet, 11 x 7 Baking Dish

2 Cups Kidney Beans, cooked
4 Cups Turkey Breast, cooked and shredded
3/4 Cup Red Pepper, chopped
1/2 Cup Orange Pepper, chopped
3 Cups Escarole, chopped
1 Tablespoon Chili Powder
1 teaspoon dried Oregano
1/2 teaspoon Salt
4 Roma Tomatoes, chopped
1/2 Cup Water
Nonstick Cooking Spray

Topping:
1 Cup Whole Wheat Flour
3/4 Cup Polenta or Cornmeal
1/2 teaspoon Baking Soda
1 teaspoon Honey
1 Cup Lowfat Milk
1 Large Egg

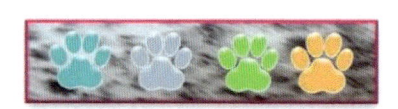

Prepare kidney beans in the electric pressure cooker ahead of time. Prepare turkey breast in electric pressure cooker. Set both aside.

Preheat oven.

Heat the large skilled over medium heat. Coat with cooking spray and sauté peppers for 5 minutes. Stir in spices and escarole, cook until wilted. Add tomatoes, kidney beans, and shredded turkey. Cook 5 more minutes.

Pour mixture into the baking dish sprayed with cooking spray.

To make topping, combine dry ingredients. Stir in honey, milk, and egg. Mix until just blended.

Spread over turkey mixture and bake for 18-20 minutes until topping is brown.

SERVING SIZE:
Makes: 6 servings
Calories per serving: 430

Human: 1 serving
Canine:
Extra Large: 1 serving
Large: 1 serving
Medium: 1/2 serving
Small: 1/4 serving

NUTRIENTS (per human serving):

Protein: 46 gm
Carbohydrate: 48 gm
Fat: 6 gm

Calcium: 102 mg
Phosphorus: 562 mg

SERVING SUGGESTIONS:
Serve with a dollop of plain nonfat yogurt or sour cream

TIPS:
Save leftover holiday turkey to use in this meal.

You can also use beef or chicken and add other vegetables or greens.

PLUS Additives:

Canine:
Extra Large: 3/4 cup turkey breast, 1 teaspoon of crushed egg shells

Large: 1/2 cup turkey breast, 1 teaspoon crushed egg shells.

Medium: 1/4 cup turkey breast, 1/4 - 1/2 teaspoon crushed egg shells.

Small: 1/8 cup turkey breast, 1/8 - 1/4 teaspoon crushed egg shells.

Humans: Sprinkle with garlic and onion powder and hot pepper flakes.

Exercise: Work on some gaps in the obedience training.

LUNA SAYS:

"I like the polenta topping. I don't eat this often so it is a nice treat."

Roast Pork with Beans and Cranberries

4-PAWS

Another great one-pot meal full of nutrients. The fresh cranberries add a burst of tartness.

OVEN: N/A

EQUIPMENT: Electric Pressure Cooker

2 1/2 pound Pork Sirloin Tip Roast
1/2 teaspoon salt
1/4 teaspoon pepper
Olive Oil Spray
1 teaspoon Dried Sage
Nonstick Cooking Spray
1 Cup fresh Navy Beans
2 1/2 Cups Water
1/2 pound Frozen or Fresh Green Beans
1/2 Cup Celery, chopped
1/2 Cup Fresh Cranberries
2 Tablespoons Honey

Sprinkle pork roast with salt and pepper. Rub with sage. Spray pressure cooker with cooking spray. Insert pork roast.

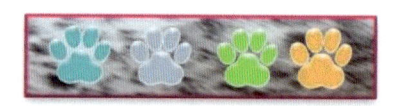

Add remaining ingredients to pressure cooker. Be sure beans are covered by the water.

Cook for 30 minutes. Let stand until pressure releases on own, about 30 minutes.

Serve warm.

SERVING SIZE:
Makes: 6 servings
Calories per serving: 367

Human: 1 serving
Canine:
Extra Large: 1 serving
Large: 1 serving
Medium: 1/2 serving
Small: 1/4 serving

NUTRIENTS (per human serving):

Protein: 52 gm
Carbohydrate: 30 gm
Fat: 4 gm

Calcium: 77 mg
Phosphorus: 595 mg

SERVING SUGGESTIONS:
Serve with rice or a flatbread PAW-ket (Page 112) for sopping up the juice.

TIPS:
Make additional pork and create small portion-size servings for freezing.

PLUS Additives:

Canine:
Extra Large: 4 ounces of pork, 1 teaspoon of crushed egg shells

Large: 3 ounces of pork, 1 teaspoon crushed egg shells.

Medium: 2 ounce of pork, 1/4 - 1/2 teaspoon crushed egg shells.

Small: 1/2 - 1 ounce of pork, 1/8 - 1/4 teaspoon crushed egg shells.

Humans: Sprinkle with garlic and onion powder.

Exercise: Reverse your walking route and add a new path or street.

LUNA SAYS:

"Not much else to say about this meal other than, Yum!"

Main ARF-Fair

MUTTball SNOOP with Greens

4-PAWS
Two kinds of greens add to the nutritional value of this soup. Very similar to Italian Wedding Soup without all the sodium.

OVEN: N/A
EQUIPMENT: Large Stockpot

Prepare Quinoa MUTTballs (Page 109).

1 Tablespoon Olive Oil
1/2 Cup Celery, chopped
1 Cup Bok Choy, chopped
1 Cup Mushrooms, chopped
6 Cups Kale, chopped
1/4 teaspoon Ground Black Pepper
1/2 teaspoon Salt
1 Cup Apple Purée
5 Cups Fresh Broth
Grated Pecorino-Romano Cheese

Heat oil in large stock pot. Sauté celery, bok choy, and mushrooms for about 5 minutes. Add kale, salt, and pepper.

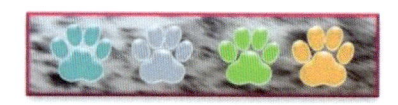

Cook for 1-2 minutes. Add remaining ingredients. Bring to a boil, cover and simmer for 10 minutes.

Add cooked Quinoa MUTTballs. Simmer for another 5 minutes until heated through.

Ladle into bowls and sprinkle with a little grated cheese.

Eat Your Own Dog Food Series

SERVING SIZE:
Makes: 6 servings
Calories per serving: 287

Human: 1 serving
Canine:
Extra Large: 2 serving
Large: 1 1/2 servings
Medium: 1 serving
Small: 1/2 serving

NUTRIENTS
(per human serving):

Protein: 21 gm
Carbohydrate: 22 gm
Fat: 13 gm

Calcium: 145 mg
Phosphorus: 299 mg

SERVING SUGGESTIONS:
Serve with half of a flatbread PAW-ket (Page 112) or an Almond ROLL-over (Page 111).

TIPS:
Make a double recipe of MUTTballs and add extra to your canine portions.

Making the MUTTballs ahead of time saves a lot of cooking time.

PLUS Additives:

Canine:
Extra Large: 7 MUTTballs, 1 teaspoon of crushed egg shells

Large: 5 MUTTballs, 1 teaspoon crushed egg shells.

Medium: 3 MUTTballs, 1/4 - 1/2 teaspoon crushed egg shells.

Small: 1-2 MUTTballs, 1/8 - 1/4 teaspoon crushed egg shells.

Humans: Sprinkle with garlic and onion powder.

Exercise: Time for another interval walk. Alternate walking for 5 minutes and then stopping to do 10 squats. Do this for the length of your usual walk.

LUNA SAYS:

"My mom sure knows how to serve us meatballs (dad and me) ?"

Main ARF-Fair

Fish CHOWDOWNner

4-PAWS
A great way to include fish in your meals. Great for shellfish too. The sweet corn taste pairs well with the Lima beans.

OVEN: N/A
EQUIPMENT: Medium Stockpot.

1 Medium Sweet Potato
8 Asparagus Spears
3 Cups of Homemade Chicken Stock
1 teaspoon salt
2 2/3 Cups Frozen Corn, thawed
1 pound of White Fish cut into 1-inch pieces
1 Cup Cooked Lima Beans
1/8 teaspoon Ground Black Pepper
1 Cup Apple Purée
1 Cup Lowfat Milk
1 Tablespoon Arrowroot Starch

Cook lima beans ahead of time using an electric pressure cooker.

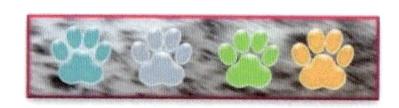

Core, chop, and purée 2 red apples in a food processor. Leave skin on.
Peel sweet potato and dice into 1/2 inch cubes. Clean asparagus, remove ends, and chop into 1/4-inch slices.

Add potatoes, asparagus, broth, and salt to the stockpot. Simmer for 10 minutes.

Put the corn in the food processor and pulse 4-6 times to chop. Add the corn to the stockpot and cook 5-10 minutes longer.

Add the fish, lima beans, apple puree, and pepper. simmer for 5-10 minutes until fish is cooked through.

Mix arrowroot with milk until dissolved. Add milk mixture to pot and simmer a few minutes until thick.

SERVING SIZE:
Makes: 6 servings
Calories per serving: 288

Human: 1 serving
Canine:
Extra Large: 1 serving
Large: 1 serving
Medium: 1/2 serving
Small: 1/4 serving

NUTRIENTS (per human serving):

Protein: 23 gm
Carbohydrate: 45 gm
Fat: 3 gm

Calcium: 98 mg
Phosphorus: 368 mg

SERVING SUGGESTIONS:
You could add sardines to this one instead of more fish to up the protein and fat content. No need to add the olive oil if using sardines.

TIPS:
Be sure to cook up an extra fish fillet or two to add to your canine serving. Fresh salmon works well with this chowder instead of white fish.

PLUS Additives:

Canine:
Extra Large: 1/2 - 3/4 pound fish, 1 Tablespoon olive oil, 1 teaspoon of crushed egg shells

Large: 1/4 - 1/2 pound fish, 1 Tablespoon olive oil, 1 teaspoon crushed egg shells.

Medium: 1/4 - 1/2 pound fish, 2 teaspoons olive oil, 1/4 - 1/2 teaspoon crushed egg shells.

Small: 1/8-1/4 pound fish, 1 teaspoon olive oil, 1/8 - 1/4 teaspoon crushed egg shells.

Humans: Sprinkle with garlic and onion powder.

Exercise: Time to play together with your favorite toy or a good game of fetch.

LUNA SAYS:

"I get to eat fish at least once a week. It's a nice change from all that meat."

GROWLED Buffalo Chicken Sliders

4-PAWS
A light sauce keeps these sliders tame and not too hot. Try gorgonzola cheese for a little change.

OVEN: N/A
EQUIPMENT: Small Bowl, Meat Mallet, Food Brush, Grill Pan or Large Skillet.

4 6-ounce Boneless, Skinless, Chicken Breasts
1 Tablespoons Hot Sauce
1 Tablespoon Water
2 Tablespoons Honey
Nonstick Cooking Spray

Sauce:
1/4 Cup Yogurt
1/4 Cup Pear purée
1/4 teaspoon Celery Seed

2 ounces Gorgonzola or Blue Cheese, crumbled
8 Almond-Wheat ROLL-overs

Prepare Almond-Wheat ROLL-overs (Page 111) ahead of time.

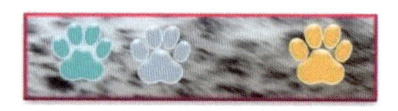

In a small bowl, combine sauce ingredients. Chill until ready to use.

Pound down chicken breasts to even thickness about 1/4 to 1/2 inch thick Cut each breast in half. Sprinkle with salt and pepper.

In a small bowl mix hot sauce, water, and honey. Brush mixture on both sides of each flattened chicken breast half.

Preheat the grill pan or skillet. Spray with cooking spray. Grill/cook chicken about 4 minutes per side. Brush on additional sauce, if desired.

Remove from heat to serving platter. Top each chicken breast with a bit of crumbled cheese

Toast rolls lightly. Place chicken on roll and top with 1 Tablespoon of sauce.

SERVING SIZE:
Makes: 4 servings (2 sliders)
Calories per serving: 281
With 1 Almond ROLL-over: 540

Human: 1 serving
Canine:
Extra Large: 1 serving
Large: 1 serving
Medium: 1/2 serving
Small: 1/4 serving

NUTRIENTS (per human serving):

Protein: 49 gm
Carbohydrate: 53 gm
Fat: 17 gm

Calcium: 42 mg
Phosphorus: 417 mg

SERVING SUGGESTIONS:
See the **SNOOPER-Bowl Sunday Party** Theme-Day ARF-Fair (Page 133).

TIPS:
Make a few extra and freeze them for later.

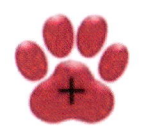

PLUS Additives:

Canine:
Extra Large: 1 chicken breasts, 1 teaspoon of crushed egg shells

Large: 3/4 chicken breast, 1 teaspoon crushed egg shells.

Medium: 1/2 - 3/4 chicken breast, 1/4 - 1/2 teaspoon crushed egg shells.

Small: 1/4-1/2 chicken breast, 1/8 - 1/4 teaspoon crushed egg shells.

Humans: Sprinkle with garlic and onion powder.

Exercise: Time for a good run at the dog park.

LUNA SAYS:

"Don't get carried away with the spice on this meal."

Faux-Ham, Sweet Potato, and Edamame Hash

4-PAWS
You will think you are eating real smoked ham. Nope, still pork, but with no chemicals, preservatives, or salt.

OVEN: N/A
EQUIPMENT: Electric Pressure Cooker, Large Skillet

2 pound Pork Sirloin Tip Roast
1/2 teaspoon Cinnamon
1/4 teaspoon Nutmeg
1/8 teaspoon Cloves
1/2 teaspoon Mustard Powder
1 Tablespoon Honey

1 pound Butternut Squash, peeled and cut into 1/4 inch cubes
1 12-ounce Package Frozen Shelled Edamame
1 1/2 Cups Frozen Corn
1/4 Cup Broth (from pork)
1 teaspoon Dried Chopped Thyme
1/2 teaspoon Salt
1/2 teaspoon Ground Pepper

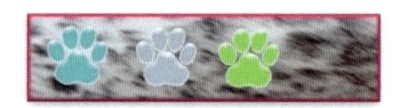

Prepare pork ahead of time using the electric pressure cooker. Rub pork with spices and drizzle with honey. Add 1-inch of water and cook for 40-minutes. When cooled and pressure reduced, dice pork into small cubes.

Heat the olive oil in the large skillet. Sauté the squash for 5 minutes. Stir in edamame, corn, broth, and thyme.

Reduce heat to medium. Cover and cook for 10 minutes, stirring occasionally, until squash is done. Stir in pork cubes, salt, and pepper.

Heat through and serve.

SERVING SIZE:
Makes: 6
Calories per serving: 336

Human: 1 serving
Canine:
Extra Large: 1 serving
Large: 1 serving
Medium: 1/2 serving
Small: 1/8 - 1/4 serving

NUTRIENTS (per human serving):

Protein: 44 gm
Carbohydrate: 28 gm
Fat: 6 gm

Calcium: 97 mg
Phosphorus: 530 mg

SERVING SUGGESTIONS:
Serve with a mixed berry fruit salad or the Mixed Greens, pear and Candied Walnut Salad (Page 96).

TIPS:
Make extra pork and freeze in portion size resealable plastic bags so you always have some on hand to add to your canine portion.

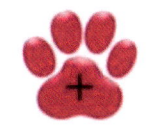

PLUS Additives:

Canine:
Extra Large: 5 ounces of pork, 1 teaspoon of crushed egg shells

Large: 4 ounces of pork, 1 teaspoon crushed egg shells.

Medium: 3 ounce of pork, 1/4 - 1/2 teaspoon crushed egg shells.

Small: 1 - 2 ounces of pork, 1/8 - 1/4 teaspoon crushed egg shells.

Humans: Sprinkle with garlic and onion powder.

Exercise: Spend 30 minutes stretching, relaxing, and meditating together.

LUNA SAYS:

"My favorite mix of spices, again."

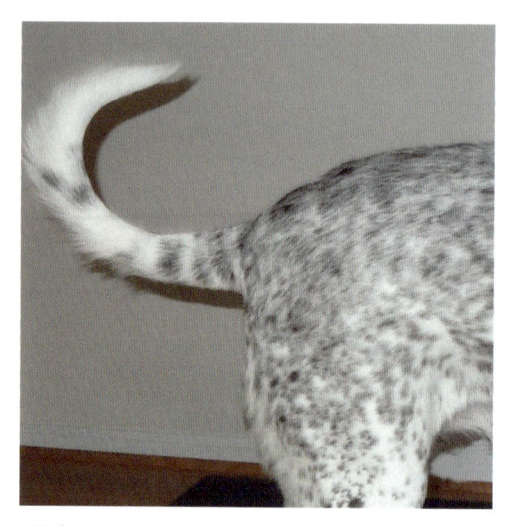

"These are sure to create a tail-waggin' experience."

Vege-TAILbles & Flanks

Your mom can use these vegetable and side dish recipes to pair nicely with some of the main ARF-Fairs to achieve the **4-PAWS.**

Or she can pair these with her own recipe for a grilled, pan-seared, or roasted meat dish. These go well with fish and salmon too.

If you have questions about any recipe contained in this book, please email your questions to us at **eatwithluna@gmail.com**.

Receive new side-dish recipes each week by joining our online community at
www.eatyourowndogfood.net

1. Asparagus-Spinach PLOPcakes   86
2. Parmesan-Zucchini Crisps   87
3. Balsamic-Roasted Carrots and Par-
   SNOOPS   88
4. Sweet Potato Chips   89
5. Cauliflower-Carrot MUSH   90
6. Quinoa and Black Beans   91
7. Split-Pea LOAFIN'   92
8. Fresh Fruit Salsa   93
9. COOL-Slaw   94
10. Drunken Green Beans   95
11. Mixed Greens, Candied Walnut, and
    Pear Salad   96
12. Vegetable PAW-ella   97

Asparagus-Spinach PLOPcakes

4-PAWS
These are great for breakfast or as a side dish for a main meal.

OVEN: N/A

EQUIPMENT: Electric Griddle or Large Skillet, Medium Bowl, Whisk

1 Cup Milk
3 Eggs
1/3 Cup Nonfat Yogurt
5 ounces of Fresh Spinach
¼ pound Asparagus, trimmed and chopped small
3 Tablespoons Grated Pecorino-Romano or Parmesan Cheese
½ teaspoon salt
¼ teaspoon pepper
½ Cup Almond Flour
Olive Oil Spray

Whisk together milk, eggs, and yogurt. Stir in spinach, asparagus, and cheese. Add flour, salt, and pepper. Mix well.

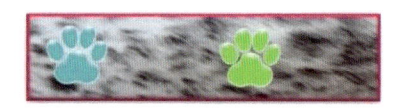

Heat griddle or skillet to medium heat. Spray with olive oil.

Pour ¼ cup of batter per cake on griddle or skillet. Cook about 2-3 minutes until golden brown and slightly puffy.

Flip over and cook another 2-3 minutes.

Spray griddle or skillet with olive oil between each batch.

SERVING SIZE:
Makes: 12 cakes
Serving: 3 pancakes
Calories per serving: 158

Human: 1 serving
Canine:
Extra Large: 1 serving
Large: 1 serving
Medium: 1/2 serving
Small: 1/8 - 1/4 serving

Parmesan-Zucchini Crisps

4-PAWS
These get crispy because of the cheese, which also adds a great flavor. These make a great snack or can be used as a side dish for a main meal.

OVEN: 450 Degrees F
EQUIPMENT: Medium Bowl, Small Bowl, Baking Sheet

1 Medium Zucchini
1 Medium Yellow Squash
1 Tablespoon Olive Oil
¼ Cup Grated Pecorino-Romano or Parmesan Cheese
¼ Cup Coconut Flour or Almond Flour
1/8 teaspoon Salt
Freshly Ground Black Pepper
Nonstick Cooking Spray

Slice the zucchini and yellow squash into ¼ inch thick rounds and place in a medium bowl. Toss with olive oil. In a small bowl, combine coconut flour and cheese, salt, and a few turns of pepper.

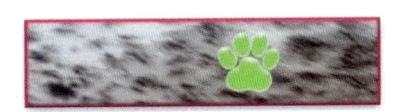

Dip each round into the flour/cheese mixture coating it evenly on both sides. Press the coating to stick.

Place rounds in a single layer on the prepared baking sheet.

Bake until crisp about 30 minutes. Remove with a spatula and serve immediately.

SERVING SIZE:
Makes: 6 servings
Serving size: 1/2 cup
Calories per serving: 105

Human: 1 serving
Canine:
Extra Large: 1 serving
Large: 3/4 - 1 serving
Medium: 1/2 serving
Small: 1/8 - 1/4 serving

Balsamic-Roasted Carrots and Par-SNOOPS

4-PAWS
Great side dish with a unique combination of sweet and sour flavors.

OVEN: 400 Degrees F
EQUIPMENT: Small and Large Bowls, Baking Sheet

1½ Pounds Carrots
1 Pound Parsnips
2 Tablespoons Agave Nectar
3 Tablespoons Balsamic Vinegar
4 Tablespoons of Olive Oil
1/2 Cup Chopped Dried Cherries (unsweetened)
¼ Cup Chopped Fresh Parsley
1 teaspoon Lemon Zest
4-oz Feta Cheese
Nonstick Cooking Spray

Preheat the oven. Peel carrots and parsnips. Cut into thin strips lengthwise about 2-3 inches long.

In a large bowl, whisk together agave nectar, vinegar, and 3 Tablespoons of olive oil. Add cut carrots and parsnips and toss to coat.

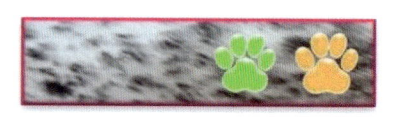

Spray the baking sheet with nonstick cooking spray. Spread the carrots and parsnips on the baking sheet and sprinkle with a little salt and pepper. Bake for 40-45 minutes or until vegetables are tender, stirring every 15 minutes while baking.

While carrots and parsnips are baking, in the small bowl, toss together 1 Tablespoon olive oil, cherries, parsley, lemon zest, and feta cheese. When carrots and parsnips are baked, transfer to a serving bowl or platter. Gently toss vegetables with feta cheese mixture. Serve warm.

SERVING SIZE:
Makes: 10 servings
Calories per serving: 186

Human: 1 serving
Canine:
Extra Large: 1/2 serving
Large: 1/2 serving
Medium: 1/4 serving
Small: 1/8 serving

Sweet Potato Chips

4-PAWS
These don't get real crispy, but the cinnamon sprinkle makes them more of a dessert than a vegetable.

OVEN: 400 Degrees F
EQUIPMENT: Medium Bowl, Small Bowl, Baking Sheet

2 Large Sweet Potatoes
Olive Oil Spray
Ground Cinnamon
Nonstick Cooking Spray

Peel the sweet potatoes and slice into ¼ inch thick rounds. Place in a medium bowl and spray and toss with enough olive oil to coat.

Spray baking sheet with nonstick cooking spray.

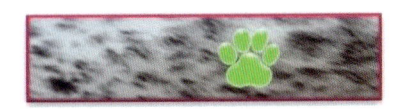

Place rounds in a single layer on the prepared baking sheet.

Bake until crisp about 30-40 minutes, stirring occasionally.

Remove from oven and sprinkle with desired amount of cinnamon.

Serve immediately.

SERVING SIZE:
Makes: 6 servings
Serving size: 1/2 cup
Calories per serving: 52

Human: 1 serving
Canine:
Extra Large: 1 serving
Large: 3/4 - 1 serving
Medium: 1/2 serving
Small: 1/4 serving

Cauliflower-Carrot MUSH

4-PAWS
A great alternative to mashed potatoes with a similar consistency.

OVEN: N/A
EQUIPMENT: Medium Saucepan, Grater, Stick Blender, Microwave Safe Container with Lid

1 Head of Fresh Cauliflower
1 Carrot, peeled and shredded
1 Tablespoon Butter
Sea Salt

Remove leaves and chop cauliflower into small, equal size florets. Place in medium saucepan with about 1" water. Cover and cook until soft and florets are easily pierced with a fork and fall apart. (Note: cauliflower can be steamed in the microwave if desired, or you can use a stovetop steamer basket.) While cauliflower is steaming, peel and rinse carrots. Shred carrots and place in a small microwave safe container. Add 1-2 Tablespoons of water. Cover and microwave for 3-5 minutes or until carrots are soft and cooked. Drain excess water.

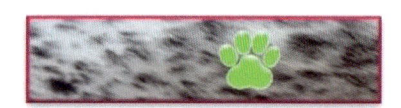

When cauliflower is steamed, drain excess water. Mash using a stick blender until smooth. Using a spoon, mix in butter and cooked shredded carrots.

Options: Add ¼ Cup Grated Pecorino-Romano or Parmesan Cheese and lightly salt (humans only: add garlic powder).

SERVING SIZE:
Makes: 4 servings
Serving size: 1/2 - 2/3 cup
Calories per serving: 85

Human: 1 serving
Canine:
Extra Large: 1 serving
Large: 1/2 serving
Medium: 1/4 serving
Small: 1/8 serving

Quinoa and Black Beans

4-PAWS
Power packed full of protein and complex carbohydrates with not all the fat. Great on its own or paired with a meat source for your canine servings.

OVEN: N/A
EQUIPMENT: Electric Pressure Cooker, Medium Saucepan

1 Teaspoon Canola Oil
¾ Cup Uncooked Quinoa
1 ½ Cups Homemade Vegetable Broth
1 teaspoon Ground Cumin
1 Cup Frozen Corn
2 Cups Cooked Black Beans
½ Cup Fresh Cilantro, chopped

Prework: Prepare black beans ahead of time using the electric pressure cooker.

Rinse quinoa. In a small saucepan, mix quinoa and vegetable broth. Season with cumin and bring to a boil. Cover, reduce heat, and simmer for 20 minutes.

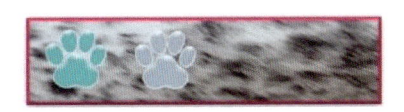

Stir in frozen corn and simmer 5 more minutes until heated through.

Mix in black beans and cilantro. Serve as a side or double the serving for a vegetarian meal.

SERVING SIZE:
Makes: 10 servings
Serving size: 1/2 - 2/3 cup
Calories per serving: 153

Human: 1 serving
Canine:
Extra Large: 1 serving
Large: 1 serving
Medium: 1/2 serving
Small: 1/8 - 1/4 serving

Split-Pea LOAFIN'

4-PAWS
Who knew you would like split peas. This is a nutritious, protein-packed, vegetable side for any main meal or your own creation.

OVEN: 325 Degrees F
EQUIPMENT: Large Skillet, Food Processor, Loaf Pan or 1-Quart Casserole Dish

2 Cups Cooked Split Peas (thick texture)
Olive Oil Spray
½ Cup Carrots, shredded
½ Cup Mushrooms, chopped
1 Cup Celery, finely diced
½ Cup Almond Flour
2 Tablespoons of Olive Oil
2 Egg Whites
1/8 teaspoon Thyme
¼ teaspoon Marjoram
Nonstick Cooking Spray

Preheat the oven.

Coat the skillet with olive oil. Sauté carrots, mushrooms, and celery over medium-high heat until soft.

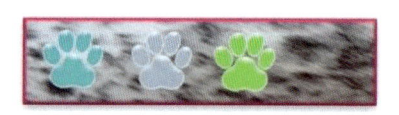

Mix all ingredients together in a food processor until smooth.

Prepare a loaf pan or 1 quart casserole dish with cooking spray. Pack mixture into the pan.

Bake for 45 minutes.

SERVING SIZE:
Makes: 8 slices
Calories per slice: 135

Human: 1 slice
Canine:
Extra Large: 1 slice
Large: 1 slice
Medium: 1/4 - 1/2 slice
Small: 1/8 - 1/4 slice

Fresh Fruit Salsa

4-PAWS
Get creative with this one. Try watermelon, pineapple, mango, or even kiwi. This is great as a topping for any main meal or your own creation.

OVEN: N/A
EQUIPMENT: Food Processor, Small Microwave Safe Bowl

3 Roma Tomatoes, chopped
1 teaspoon Jalapenos, diced
½ Cup Fruit/Vegetable (peach, pear, mango, pineapple, cucumber), chopped
1 Tablespoon Fresh Cilantro, chopped
1 Tablespoon White Vinegar
1 Tablespoon Honey
1 teaspoon Lime Juice
Fresh Ground Pepper, 2 turns

Place tomatoes, jalapenos, fruit, and cilantro in food processor. Pulse/process a few times until still slightly chunky. For smoother salsa pulse/process until desired consistency.

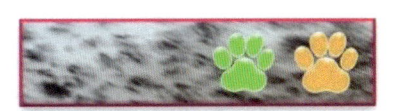

Pour salsa into a microwave safe small bowl. Mix in vinegar, honey, lime juice, and ground pepper.

Microwave for 1 minute on high setting. Refrigerate for 1 hour.

Serve as a topping for grilled chicken or fish, or a topping for an omelet.

SERVING SIZE:
Makes: 1 cup of salsa
Serving size: 1/4 cup
Calories per serving: 50

Human: 1 serving
Canine:
Extra Large: 1 serving
Large: 1/2 serving
Medium: 1/4 serving
Small: 1/8 serving

COOL-Slaw

4-PAWS
Cauliflower adds a new twist to traditional cole slaw. See for yourself; it is hard to tell the difference. Nonfat yogurt keeps the fat and sugar lower.

OVEN: N/A
EQUIPMENT: Food Processor, Small and Medium Bowls

1 Head of Cauliflower
2 Carrots, grated
1/4 Cup Green Pepper, finely grated
1 Cup Nonfat Yogurt
2 Tablespoons Olive Oil
2 Tablespoons Dijon Mustard
1 Tablespoon Cider Vinegar
1 Tablespoon Lemon Juice
1 Tablespoon Honey
1/4 teaspoon Celery Seed
2 Tablespoons Heavy Whipping Cream

Clean and chop the cauliflower into small florets. Place cauliflower in food processor and pulse until it looks like the consistency of rice or coarsely chopped cabbage.

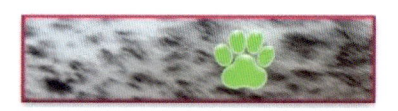

Place cauliflower in the medium bowl. Stir in grated carrots and diced green peppers.

In the small bowl, mix remaining ingredients (yogurt through whipping cream).

Add to cauliflower mixture toss gently to mix. Chill for 2 hours or overnight before serving.

SERVING SIZE:
Makes: 6 servings
Serving size: 1/2 cup
Calories per serving: 120

Human: 1 serving
Canine:
Extra Large: 1 serving
Large: 1/2 serving
Medium: 1/4 serving
Small: 1/8 serving

Drunken Green Beans

4-PAWS
These are simmered in broth to give them flavor and create that overcooked, "sloshed" texture we remember.

OVEN: N/A
EQUIPMENT: Medium Saucepan

1 pound of Frozen Green Beans
1 Cup Pork Broth (or other type)
1/4 Cup Mushrooms
1/4 Cup Almonds, finely chopped
1/4 teaspoon Ground Black Pepper
1/4 teaspoon Salt

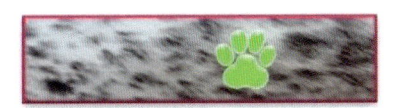

Place all ingredients in the sauce pan. Simmer over low heat until green beans are soft, about 15-20 minutes.

SERVING SIZE:
Makes: 6 servings
Serving size: 1/2 - 2/3 cup
Calories per serving: 40

Human: 1 serving
Canine:
Extra Large: 1 serving
Large: 1 serving
Medium: 1/2 serving
Small: 1/8 - 1/4 serving

Mixed Greens, Candied Walnut, and Pear Salad

4-PAWS
Pair this with any main meal for added greens and fruit. The slight sweetness on the walnuts is an added treat.

OVEN: N/A
EQUIPMENT: Small Nonstick Skillet, Small Bowl, Whisk, Large Salad Bowl

2/3 Cup Walnuts
1 Tablespoon Honey
2 Tablespoons Balsamic Vinegar
1 1/2 teaspoons Dijon Mustard
3 Tablespoons Olive Oil
8 Cups Mixed Greens or Artisan Lettuce Mix, torn
1 Pear, ripe and thinly sliced
1/4 teaspoon Ground Black Pepper

Toast walnuts in the small skillet over medium heat. When toasted, add the honey and stir a few minutes until walnuts are coated. Be careful not to burn the walnuts. Let cool.

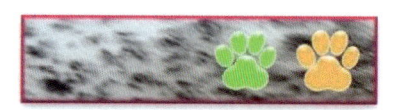

Combine vinegar and mustard using a whisk. Gradually whisk in olive oil and pepper.

Place lettuce in a bowl, top with sliced pears and toasted walnuts. Drizzle dressing over salad. Toss slightly and then serve.

SERVING SIZE:
Makes 8 servings
Serving size: 1 cup
Calories per serving: 170

Human: 1 serving
Canine:
Extra Large: 1/2 serving
Large: 1/2 serving
Medium: 1/4 serving
Small: 1/8 serving

Vegetable PAW-ella

4-PAWS

Flavorful side or larger dinner portion. Be sure to add meat for your canine servings.

OVEN: N/A
EQUIPMENT: Electric Pressure Cooker (See note.)

1 Cup Green Peppers, chopped
1 Cup Mushrooms, chopped
1 Cup Roma Tomatoes, chopped
1/2 Cup Dried Figs, chopped
1 Cup Frozen Artichoke Hearts, thawed and coarsely chopped
½ Cup Frozen Green Peas
1 ½ Cups Uncooked Brown Rice
1 Cups Homemade Chicken Broth
2 Cups Water
½ teaspoon Ground Turmeric
¼ teaspoon Ground Thyme
1 Tablespoon Fresh Chopped Parsley
¼ teaspoon Ground Pepper

Combine all ingredients in the electric pressure cooker and cook using the Rice setting.

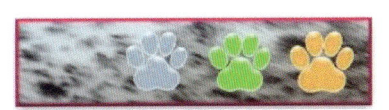

Let sit for 30-45 minutes until pressure releases and you can open the pressure cooker.

Serve warm.

NOTE: If using a stockpot, sauté peppers and mushrooms in a little olive oil. Stir in rice, figs, broth, water, turmeric and thyme. Bring to a boil, reduce heat, cover and simmer about 30 minutes. Stir in tomatoes, artichoke hearts, peas, parsley, and pepper. Cover and cook for 15 minutes or until liquid is absorbed and rice is tender.

SERVING SIZE:

Makes 10 servings
Serving size: 1 cup
Calories per serving: 175

Human: 1 serving
Canine:
Extra Large: 1 serving
Large: 3/4 serving
Medium: 1/2 serving
Small: 1/8 - 1/4 serving

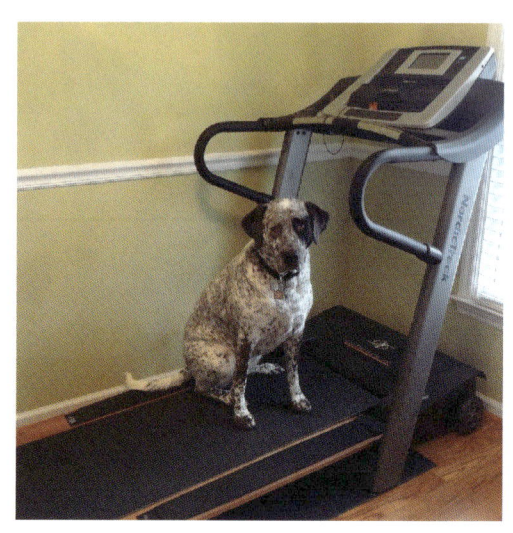

"Mom, I'm ready for my afternoon run."

Nibbles & PAW-Food

Your mom can start your PAWs-itively satisfying experience off with one of these little snacks or finger-foods (AKA PAW-food).

These are great afternoon snacks and will give you more energy for your afternoon workout.

If you have questions about any recipe contained in this book, please email your questions to us at **eatwithluna@gmail.com**.

Receive new treat recipes each week by joining our online community at
www.eatyourowndogfood.net

1. Homemade GROWLnola   100
2. Jelly-Belly-Donut Muffins   102
3. Sesame Crackers   104
4. Faux-Sausage Bites   105
5. Rip the Stuffins Out Muffins   106
6. Brown Rice WAGGIN' Waffles   108
7. Quinoa MUTTballs   109
8. Peanut Butter Hummus   110
9. Almond-Wheat Roll-OVERs   111
10. Homemade Flat Bread PAW-kets   112

Eat Your Own Dog Food Series

Homemade GROWLnola Cereal

4-PAWS

Looks are deceiving. A little goes a long way here. This power-packed treat can be used as a cereal or topping for yogurt or used as a topping for a fruit crisp.

OVEN: 250 Degrees F
EQUIPMENT: Large and Small Bowls, 11 x 17 Roasting Pan or Baking Sheet

1 ¼ Cup Rolled Oats
1/3 Cup Sesame Seeds
1/3 Cup Wheat Bran
¼ Cup Soy Flour
¼ Cup Non-Fat Dry Milk
¼ Cup of Ground Flaxmeal
¼ Cup Chopped Almonds
¼ Cup Toasted Sunflower Seeds
¼ Cup Chopped Pecans
¼ Cup Canola Oil
¼ Cup Honey
¼ Cup Chopped Dried Cherries (No Sugar added)
¼ Cup Chopped Figs or Dates

___

Preheat the oven. Combine all dry ingredients and nuts in a large mixing bowl.

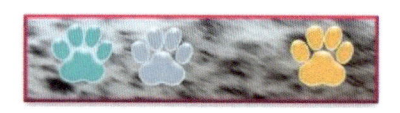

Combine honey and oil in a small bowl or large liquid measuring cup. Pour oil and honey mixture over dry ingredients and fold in with a large spoon until all dry ingredients are well coated.

Pour mixture in to roasting pan and distribute evenly in the pan.

Bake for at least 1 hour stirring every 10-15 minutes. Stir in the dried fruit during the last 10 minutes of baking time. The mixture should turn light brown in color. Additional baking time may be needed.

Cool thoroughly and store in an airtight container in a cool place for about 3-4 weeks.

Refrigerate for longer storage.

SERVING SIZE:
Makes 1 Quart
Serving size: 1/4 cup
Calories per serving: 165

Human: 1/4 cup
Canine:
Extra Large: 1/4 cup
Large: 1/4 cup
Medium: 1/8 cup
Small: 1 Tablespoon

SERVING SUGGESTIONS:
This makes a great cereal snack with a little milk.

TIPS:
Vary your fruit and nut combinations for different flavors.

Be sure to use only dried fruit with no added sugar.

Jelly-Belly-Donut Muffins

4-PAWS
A great faux-jelly donut high in protein, complex carbohydrates, and fruit without all the sugar. Soy flour and cottage cheese provide additional nutrient value.

OVEN: 325 Degrees F
EQUIPMENT: Medium Bowl, 12-Cup Muffin Pan

¼ Cup Soy Flour
¾ Cup Brown Rice Flour
2 teaspoons Baking Powder
1 Large Egg
2 Tablespoons Canola Oil
¼ Cup Honey
½ Cup Buttermilk
½ Cup Cottage Cheese

1 Cup Frozen Mixed Berries
1 teaspoon of Agave Nectar
1 teaspoon Arrowroot Starch (for thickening)

Place frozen berries in a small sauce pan. Heat until thawed smashing berries to create more juice.

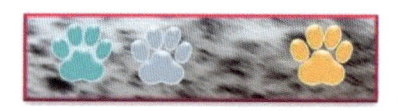

Add agave nectar and bring to a light boil. In a small measuring cup, stir arrowroot into just enough water to dissolve it. Mix until smooth.

Add to boiling berries and stir until mixture thickens and turns shiny. Set aside and cool slightly.

Combine dry ingredients. Add egg, oil, honey, buttermilk, and cottage cheese. Mix until blended.

Spray muffin pan with cooking spray. Split batter evenly between the 12 muffin cups.

Spoon 1 heaping Tablespoon of the cooled fruit mixture on top of the batter in each cup.

Using a knife, swirl/marble the fruit in each cup.

Bake for 25-30 minutes until lightly browned and a knife inserted comes out clean.

Cool for 5 minutes and remove from pan. Cool on wire rack.

SERVING SIZE:
Makes 12 muffins
Serving size: 1 muffin
Calories per serving: 125

Human: 1 muffin
Canine:
Extra Large: 1 muffin
Large: 1 muffin
Medium: 1/2 muffin
Small: 1/8 - 1/4 muffin

SERVING SUGGESTIONS:
These make great breakfast treats in the morning.

TIPS:
Add 1/2 Tablespoon of white vinegar in 1/2 cup of milk for buttermilk. Let stand for a few minutes.

Use whole grain flour to thicken if you do not have arrowroot starch.

These muffins freeze well.

Eat Your Own Dog Food Series

Sesame Crackers

4-PAWS
These go great with Peanut Butter Hummus (Page 110). Add cheese and spices such as rosemary to create new flavors.

OVEN: 400 Degrees F
EQUIPMENT: Baking Sheet, Rolling Pin, Parchment Paper, Pastry Brush

2 Cups Whole Grain Flour
1 teaspoon Baking Powder
½ teaspoon salt (optional)
½ Cup Chopped Toasted Sunflower Seeds or Nuts
1/3 Cup Olive Oil
2/3 Cup Warm Water

1 Egg White Plus 2 Tablespoons Water

Combine dry ingredients. Stir in oil and water. Mix until a smooth dough forms. Add a little more water if needed.

Divide dough in half. Cut 2 sheets of parchment paper to fit the size of your baking sheet.

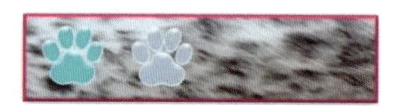

Roll out each piece of dough into a thin square or rectangular shape on the parchment paper or press flat with fingers. Dough should be rolled to 1/16" thickness. Use a sharp knife or pizza cutter to cut the dough into small 1" squares.

Brush lightly with egg white wash or spray lightly with olive oil.

Bake for 10-12 minutes until crackers are golden and crispy. Let cool and sit out overnight to establish crispness. Store in airtight container. Refrigerate for extended storage.

SERVING SIZE:
Makes approx. 48 crackers
Serving size: 4 crackers
Calories per serving: 140

Human: 1 serving
Canine:
Extra Large: 1 serving
Large: 3/4 serving
Medium: 1/2 serving
Small: 1/4 serving

104   Say "NO" to Dog Food

Faux-Sausage Bites

4-PAWS
These can be spiced as breakfast or italian. Great high protein snack.

OVEN: N/A
EQUIPMENT: Large Bowl, Nonstick or Cast Iron Skillet

2 pounds of Ground Beef (or Pork or combination)
Cooking Spray

For Italian Sausage:
¾ teaspoon Salt
¼ teaspoon Ground Black Pepper
1 Tablespoon Ground Paprika
2 Tablespoons Olive Oil
¼ teaspoon Anise Seed
¼ teaspoon Fennel Seed, Grind Anise & Fennel in a spice grinder

For Breakfast Sausage:
2 teaspoons Dried Sage
¾ teaspoon Salt
1 teaspoon Ground Black Pepper
¼ teaspoon Dried Marjoram

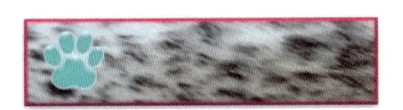

1 Tablespoon Honey
1 pinch Ground Cloves
2 Tablespoons Olive Oil

Place meat in the large bowl.

For either type, mix all spices together in a small bowl. Add spice mix and olive oil to meat. Mix until well blended.

To blend flavors, refrigerate overnight. Shape into small 2-3 inch flat round patties about ¼" thick and sauté in the nonstick or cast iron skillet until done, about 5 minutes per side.

SERVING SIZE:
Makes 20 patties
Serving size: 3 patties
Calories per serving: 146

Human: 1 serving
Canine:
Extra Large: 1 serving
Large: 1 serving
Medium: 1/2 serving
Small: 1/3 serving

Rip-the-Stuffins-Out Muffins

4-PAWS
Power-packed and great-tasting snack that tastes and feels like comfort food.

OVEN: 350 Degrees F
EQUIPMENT: Large Mixing Bowl, Medium Skillet, 12-Cup Muffin Pan

1 Loaf of Honey Whole Grain Bread (from your bread machine or fresh from a bakery; do not use prepackaged bread)

¾ Cup Chopped Red Peppers
¾ Cup Chopped Green Peppers
1 Cup Chopped Mushroom
5 Ounces Baby Spinach
6 Large Eggs
1 ½ Cups Milk
1 Tablespoon Dijon Mustard
¼ teaspoon Salt
¼ teaspoon Pepper
¾ Cup Shredded Pepper Jack Cheese (can use cheddar or another type of cheese)
Nonstick Cooking Spray
Olive Oil Spray

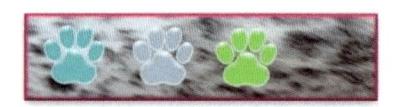

Preheat the oven. Spray muffin pan. Cut enough bread into small ½ inch cubes to make about 4 cups. Set aside.

Heat the medium skillet over medium-high heat. Coat with olive oil. Sauté both peppers and mushrooms until soft. Add spinach and cook until wilted about 1 minute. Set aside and cool slightly.

In a large bowl, whisk together eggs, milk, mustard, salt, and pepper. Stir in vegetable mixture and cheese, and then gently fold in bread cubes.

Let mixture stand for 15 minutes.

Divide mixture evenly between 12 muffin cups. Bake for 20-25 minutes until puffy and lightly browned.

Let stand for 5 minutes before removing from muffin pan.

Use a knife if necessary to loosen edges.

Serve warm.

SERVING SIZE:
Makes 12 muffins
Serving size: 1 muffin
Calories per serving: 120

Human: 1 serving
Canine:
Extra Large: 1 serving
Large: 1 serving
Medium: 1/2 serving
Small: 1/4 serving

SERVING SUGGESTIONS:
These are great any time, not just for breakfast

TIPS:
Mix it up and try different vegetable and cheese combinations.

Brown Rice WAGGIN' Waffles

4-PAWS
These make great treats with a dab of peanut butter hummus (Page 110), honey, maple syrup or homemade fruit purée.

OVEN: N/A
EQUIPMENT: Waffle Iron (standard size)

1 ¼ cups Brown Rice Flour
½ cup Almond Flour
¼ cup Brown Flaxseed Meal
2 teaspoons Baking Powder
¼ cup Canola Oil
1 Tablespoon of Honey
2 Large Eggs (beaten)
1 2/3 cups Milk
Nonstick Cooking Spray

In a large bowl, combine all the flours, flaxseed meal, and baking powder. Add oil, honey, eggs and milk. Mix until batter is smooth.

Preheat waffle iron. Pour about ¾ cup of batter onto a heated waffle iron sprayed with cooking spray or use the amount specified for your waffle iron. You may need to adjust the amount of batter to fit your waffle iron. Bake for about 3-4 minutes or as instructed for your waffle iron.

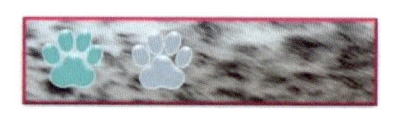

Belgian waffles require more batter and longer cooking time. Serving size and calories per serving will differ from that indicated.

Serve warm.
Great for freezing. Use toaster oven for reheating.

SERVING SIZE:
Makes 8 waffles
Serving Size: 1/2 waffle
Calories per serving: 110

Human: 1 serving
Canine:
Extra Large: 1 serving
Large: 1/2 serving
Medium: 1/2 serving
Small: 1/4 serving

Eat Your Own Dog Food Series

Quinoa MUTTballs

4-PAWS
Make a ton of these and freeze them so you always have some on hand for a quick treat/snack or to add more protein to your canine servings.

OVEN: 450 Degrees F
EQUIPMENT: Large Bowl, Small Saucepan, Baking Sheet

½ Cup Washed Quinoa
1 Pound of Ground Meat
2 Large Eggs
½ teaspoon Black Pepper
½ teaspoon Paprika
½ teaspoon Oregano
½ teaspoon Dried Parsley
Nonstick Cooking Spray

In the small saucepan, add washed quinoa to 1 cup of water and bring to a boil.

Reduce heat to low, cover, and cook about 15 minutes until water is absorbed.

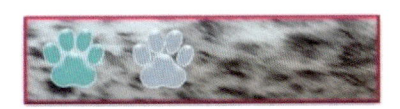

Preheat the oven.

Combine meat, eggs, spices, and cooked quinoa in a bowl. Mix until well blended.

Shape into round 1 ½ inch balls (24). Place balls on a baking sheet coated with cooking spray.

Bake for about 12-15 minutes until slightly brown.

SERVING SIZE:
Makes 24 meatballs
Serving size: 4 meatballs
Calories per serving: 200

Human: 1 serving
Canine:
Extra Large: 1 serving
Large: 1 serving
Medium: 1/2 serving
Small: 1/8 - 1/4 serving

Nibbles & PAW-Food

Peanut Butter Hummus

4-PAWS
This takes plain peanut butter to a new level: less fat and more nutritious. Pair with a Flatbread PAW-ket (Page 112) or Sesame Crackers (Page 104).

OVEN: N/A
EQUIPMENT: Electric Pressure Cooker, Food Processor

3 Tablespoons of Organic Peanut Butter (no sugar added)
1 Tablespoon Lemon Juice
1 ½ Tablespoons Olive Oil
½ teaspoon black pepper
3/8 teaspoon salt
1 ½ Cups Cooked Chickpeas
¼ Cup Water

Cook raw chickpeas in a pressure cooker (canned chickpeas contain too much sodium).

When cool enough to handle, add chickpeas to bowl of food processor.

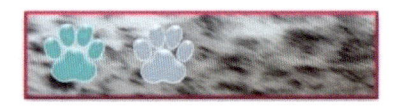

Microwave peanut butter in a small-microwave safe bowl for 20 seconds.

Add peanut butter, lemon juice, olive oil, pepper, and salt to the chickpeas in the food processor. Slowly add water while running the processor; add enough water until smooth.

Serve with sesame crackers, flat bread PAW-kets, or vegetables.

Refrigerate in airtight container.

SERVING SIZE:
Makes 8 (2 Tablespoon) servings
Calories per serving: 93

Human: 1 serving
Canine:
Extra Large: 1 serving
Large: 1 serving
Medium: 1/2 serving
Small: 1/4 serving

Almond-Wheat Roll-OVERs

4-PAWS
Another great treat on its own or paired with a main meal. These make great sliders.

OVEN: 350 Degrees F
EQUIPMENT: Bread Machine, Medium Bowl, 13 x 9 Baking Pan

1 ¾ Cup Water
2 teaspoons Salt
3 Tablespoons Olive Oil
1/3 Cup Honey
3 ½ Cups Whole Wheat Flour or Hard White Wheat Flour
1 Cups Almond Flour
2 ½ teaspoons Yeast
2 Tablespoons of Vital Wheat Gluten (Optional: makes dough more elastic and pliable)
Cooking Spray

Place all ingredients into your bread machine and use DOUGH setting.
When complete, remove dough and place in an olive oil coated bowl.

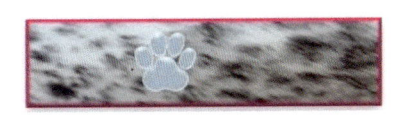

Cover bowl with a clean towel and place in a warm, draft-free location for about 30 minutes or until doubled in size.

Place on lightly floured surface and divide into 20 equal pieces and shape into balls. Place in the baking pan coated with cooking spray. Cover and let rise 30-40 minutes until doubled in size.

Bake in preheated oven for 25 minutes, or until golden brown.

SERVING SIZE:
Makes 20 rolls
Calories per roll: 130

Human: 1 rolls
Canine:
Extra Large: 1 roll
Large: 1 roll
Medium: 1/2 roll
Small: 1/4 roll

Homemade Flatbread PAW-kets

4-PAWS
Power packed snack that tastes great on its own.

OVEN: N/A
EQUIPMENT: Bread Machine, Medium Bowl, Electric Griddle

1 Cup Warm Water
1 ½ Tablespoons Olive Oil
1 ¾ teaspoons Salt
2 ¾ Cups Whole Grain Flour
2 ½ teaspoons of yeast
2 Tablespoons Vital Wheat Gluten (Optional: for elasticity)

Add ingredients to the bread machine in the above order. Use the DOUGH cycle of your bread machine.

Remove dough from the machine and place in bowl coated with olive oil.

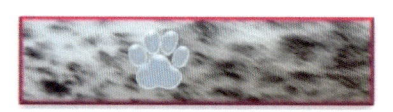

Cover with a towel and let dough rest about 30-40 minutes in a warm draft-free location.

Remove dough from bowl and place on floured work surface. Cut dough into 8 equal pieces. Form each piece into a ball with a smooth top. Place dough balls back into bowl, cover and let rest again for 30 minutes.

Preheat griddle to 350 degrees (medium-high heat). On a floured work surface flatten each dough ball with fingers to form a flat, round bread about ¼" thick. Let flattened dough rest for 5 minutes before cooking. Spray the griddle with olive oil. Cook the flat bread on the griddle for about 3-5 minutes until it begins to puff and the bottom is brown. Spray top side with olive oil, flip over and cook 3-5 minutes on the other side.

If desired, cut flatbread into 2 halves and using a small knife, carefully slice/spread open like a pita bread.

SERVING SIZE:
Makes 8 flatbreads
Calories per flatbread: 187

Human: 1 flatbread
Canine:
Extra Large: 1/2 flatbread
Large: 1/2 flatbread
Medium: 1/4 flatbread
Small: 1/8 flatbread

SERVING SUGGESTIONS:
Use for PAWed Pork (Page 68), Sloppy Lentils (Page 70), or fill with Peanut Butter Hummus (Page 110).

TIPS:
Make a ton of these ahead of time and freeze them.

When ready to serve, pop in the toaster oven set on medium setting. No need to thaw first. They come out warm and slightly crispy on the outside.

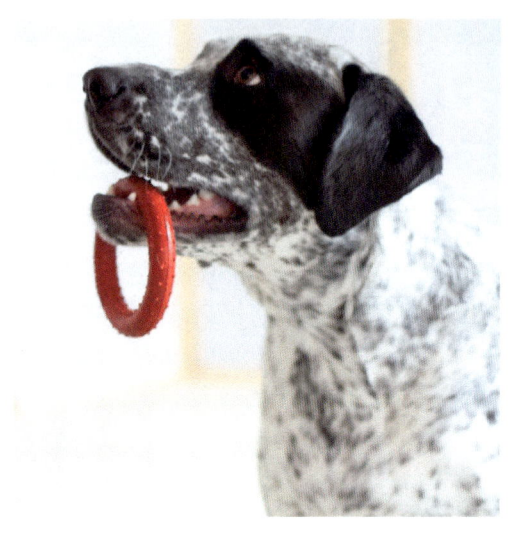

"I'll trade you a toy for an extra dollop of I'm Whupped Cream."

InDOGences

Your mom can end your dining and sharing experience with a dessert indulgence sure to achieve a chop-licking response.

Remember, everything in moderation, though.

If you have questions about any recipe contained in this book, please email your questions to us at **eatwithluna@gmail.com**.

Receive new dessert recipes each week by joining our online community at
www.eatyourowndogfood.net

1. Blueberry Yogurt Cake — 116
2. HOWL-wiian Shortcake with "I'm Whupped" Cream — 118
3. Banana Custard Pie — 120
4. Lemon Apricot Quinoa PUPcakes — 122
5. "Who Said Dogs Don't Like Fruit" Custard Treat — 123
6. Pear and Apple Galette with Olive Oil Crust — 124
7. Coconut MacaLunas — 126
8. Rice Pudding with Dates — 127
9. Cabbage Carrot Cake with Honey Cream Cheese — 128
10. Lip-Licking-Lemon Cheesecake Bites — 130

Blueberry Yogurt Cake

4-PAWS
A great balance of protein from the yogurt and high-complex carbohydrates. The fruit and touch of honey add just enough sweetness.

OVEN: 325 Degrees F
EQUIPMENT: Medium and Small Bowls, 8-inch Square Baking Dish

1/2 Cup Canola Oil
1/2 Cup Honey
2 Large Eggs
1 teaspoon Vanilla Extract
1 1/4 Cups Hard White Wheat Flour
1 teaspoon Baking Powder
1/2 teaspoon Baking Soda
1/2 Cup Plain Nonfat Yogurt
1 Cup Blueberries (fresh or thawed frozen berries)
Nonstick Cooking Spray

Topping:
1/4 Cup Honey
1 teaspoon Cinnamon
1/2 teaspoon Nutmeg
1 Cup Chopped Pecans or Walnuts

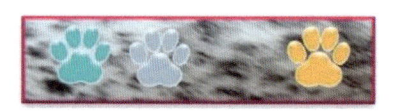

Preheat the oven. Spray baking dish with nonstick cooking spray.

In the medium bowl, mix oil and honey until blended. Beat in eggs and vanilla extract.

Add flour, baking powder, and baking soda until fully mixed, and then mix in yogurt. Gently stir in blueberries.

In the small bowl, stir together honey, cinnamon, nutmeg, and chopped nuts.

Pour half the cake batter into the prepared baking pan. Sprinkle with half of the nut topping mixture. Top with remaining batter and sprinkle with remaining topping.

Bake about 40-45 minutes until toothpick or knife inserted into center comes out clean.

Serve warm or fully cooled.

SERVING SIZE:
Makes 9 servings
Calories per serving: 390

Human: 1 serving
Canine:
Extra Large: 1/2 serving
Large: 1/4 - 1/2 serving
Medium: 1/4 - 1/8 serving
Small: 1/8 serving

SERVING SUGGESTIONS:
Serve warm with 1 Tablespoon of "I'm Whupped Cream" (Page 118) or place in a bowl with milk (Dad likes it this way).

TIPS:
Make a few of these ahead of time for freezing. Slice into portions, wrap individually in plastic wrap and freeze.

Great for dessert or for breakfast.

Use whole grain flour if unable to find hard white wheat flour.

Try other fruit and nut mixes.

Eat Your Own Dog Food Series

HOWL-wiian Shortcake with "I'm Whupped" Cream

4-PAWS
The coconut gives this shortcake great flavor and texture.

OVEN: 450 & 325 Degrees F
EQUIPMENT: Baking Sheet, Small and Medium Bowls, 9-inch Round Cake Pan

Fruit:
1 Medium Pineapple, peeled and cored
Nonstick Cooking Spray
1 Tablespoon Honey
2 Tablespoons Water
1/2 teaspoon Ground Ginger
1/8 teaspoon Ground Cloves

Shortcake:
1 1/2 Cups Hard White Wheat Flour
3/4 Cup Flaked Unsweetened Coconut
1 teaspoon baking powder
1/4 teaspoon salt
2/3 Cup Honey
1/4 Cup Canola Oil
2 Large Egg Whites
1/4 teaspoon Vanilla Extract
1/2 Cup 1% Low fat Milk

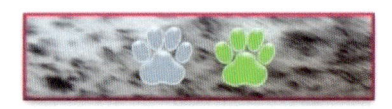

"I'm Whupped" Cream:
1 Cup Heavy Whipping cream
1-2 Tablespoons of Honey
1 teaspoon Vanilla Extract

Preheat oven to 450 Degrees F
Fruit:
Cut Pineapple into 1/2 inch slices. Arrange in a single layer on a baking sheet sprayed with nonstick cooking spray.

In the small bowl, combine honey, water, ginger, and cloves. Drizzle over pineapple. Bake for 20 minutes until lightly browned. Set aside.

Shortcake:
Decrease oven temperature to 325 Degrees F.

In a medium bowl, combine honey, oil, egg whites, vanilla and milk. Add all dry ingredients and stir until just blended. Do not over mix. Pour into cake pan sprayed with cooking spray.

118   Say "NO" to Dog Food

Bake for 35 minutes or until a toothpick inserted in center comes out clean.

Cool on wire rack in pan for 10 minutes before removing. Completely cool before assembling.

Cream:
In a metal bow, beat all whipped cream ingredients with an electric mixer or stick blender until thick.

To assemble, slice cake in half horizontally using a serrated knife. Place bottom layer on plate. Top with pineapple, whipped cream and top cake layer. Serve.

SERVING SIZE:
Makes 10 servings
Calories per serving: 300

Human: 1 slice
Canine:
Extra Large: 1/2 serving
Large: 1/4 - 1/2 serving
Medium: 1/4 - 1/8 serving
Small: 1/8 serving

SERVING SUGGESTIONS:
Serve warm if desired or use a different berry or fruit.

Banana Custard Pie

4-PAWS
All I can say is "Yum!" The thick custard is flavored with fresh bananas. This dessert is sure to go quickly.

OVEN: 350 Degrees F
EQUIPMENT: Medium and Large Bowls, Rolling Pin, Parchment Paper, 9-inch Pie Pan

Crust:
¾ Cup Hard White Wheat Flour
¼ Cup Almond Flour
1 teaspoon Ground Cinnamon
½ teaspoon Salt
¼ Cup Canola Oil
4 Tablespoons of Cold Water
Nonstick Cooking Spray

Filling:
4 Bananas
3 Eggs
2/3 Cup Milk
¼ Cup Honey
1 teaspoon Vanilla Extract
3 Tablespoons Almond Flour

Preheat oven. Spray 9" pie pan lightly with cooking spray.

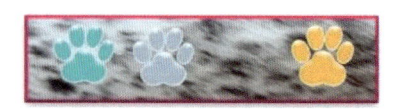

Crust: In a medium bowl, mix together flours, cinnamon, and salt. Cut in oil with a fork until flour mixture is moistened and resembles small lumps/crumbs.

Add water and mix until dough forms. Add more water one Tablespoon at a time, as necessary.

Roll dough into a 9-10 inch circle on lightly floured parchment paper. Gently flip parchment paper over and place crust in pie pan. Remove parchment paper and lightly press crust into pan and finish edges. Remove excess crust from edges if needed. Bake empty crust for 10 minutes.

Custard: While the crust is baking, in a large bowl, combine 2 crushed bananas, eggs, milk, honey, vanilla, and almond flour. Blend until creamy. Slice the remaining 2 bananas into thin slices.

Assembling Pie: When the crust is finished, place 1 layer of sliced bananas in the crust. Pour about ½ of the custard on top of banana layer.

Place another layer of sliced bananas and then remaining custard. Be sure bananas are covered by custard.

Bake for 30 minutes until custard is set. Let cool completely. Refrigerate for 1 hour before serving.

SERVING SIZE:
Makes 8 servings
Calories per serving: 300

Human: 1 serving
Canine:
Extra Large: 1/2 serving
Large: 1/4 - 1/2 serving
Medium: 1/4 - 1/8 serving
Small: 1/8 serving

SERVING SUGGESTIONS:
Decorate with "I'm Whupped" Cream (Page 118) and more banana slices, if desired.

Lemon Apricot Quinoa PUPcakes

4-PAWS
Great make-ahead snacks to have on hand. The quinoa gives these a unique flavor. Use other dried fruits to mix it up.

OVEN: 325 Degrees F
EQUIPMENT: Medium Bowl, 12-Cup Muffin Pan, Muffin Liners

1 3/4 Cup Hard White Wheat Flour
2 teaspoons baking powder
1/2 Cup Honey
3/4 Cup Lowfat Milk
3 Tablespoons Canola Oil
1 Large Egg
1 Tablespoon Lemon Zest
1 Tablespoon Lemon Juice
1 teaspoon Vanilla Extract
1 Cup Cooked Quinoa
2/3 Cup Dried Apricots, chopped

Preheat oven.
Mix flour and baking powder in a medium bowl.

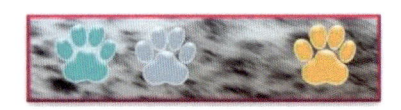

Add honey, milk, oil, egg, lemon zest, lemon juice, and vanilla. Stir until just blended. Fold in quinoa.

Split chopped apricots into 12-piles.

Line muffin pan. Pour batter into muffin liners splitting equally between the 12-cups. Place chopped apricots on top of batter in each cup.

Bake for 30 minutes or until a toothpick inserted in center come out clean.

Remove and cool on wire rack.

SERVING SIZE:
Makes 12 muffins
Serving size: 1 muffin
Calories per serving: 120

Human: 1 serving
Canine:
Extra Large: 1 serving
Large: 1 serving
Medium: 1/2 serving
Small: 1/8 - 1/4 serving

"Who Said Dogs Don't Like Fruit" Custard Treat

4-PAWS
Fresh strawberries work best for this custard treat that is sure to please.

OVEN: 350 Degrees F
EQUIPMENT: Electric Mixer or Stick Blender, Shallow 2-Quart Baking Dish.

½ pound of thinly sliced fruit or berries (strawberries, peaches, mixed berries)
4 Large eggs
1/3 Cup honey
1 Cup milk
6 Tablespoons Whole Wheat Flour
1 teaspoon Vanilla Extract
1 teaspoon Lemon Zest
1 teaspoon Lemon Juice
¼ teaspoon Cinnamon

Preheat the oven and coat the baking dish with cooking spray. Peel/rinse/slice berries or fruit and arrange in baking dish.

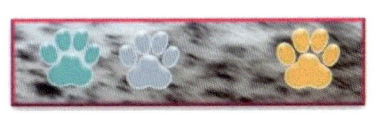

Using an electric blender, beat eggs and honey until smooth about 1-2 minutes.

Mix in milk and flour while blending on low setting. Add remaining ingredients and mix until blended.

Pour over berries and bake about 40 minutes or until puffy, set, and golden brown.

Cool before serving. Serve with a dollop of "I'm Whupped" Cream (Page 118).

SERVING SIZE:
Makes 8 servings
Serving size: 1 slice
Calories per serving: 120

Human: 1 serving
Canine:
Extra Large: 1 serving
Large: 1 serving
Medium: 1/2 serving
Small: 1/8 - 1/4 serving

Blueberry - Peach Galette with Olive Oil Crust

4-PAWS
Great, quick alternative to making a large fruit pie. The olive oil crust is easy to make.

OVEN: 425 to 350 Degrees F
EQUIPMENT: Baking Sheet, Parchment Paper, Rolling Pin, Small and Medium Bowls, Pastry Brush

Crust:
1 Cup Hard White Wheat Flour
1/2 teaspoon salt
1/4 Cup Canola Oil
3 Tablespoons Water

Filling:
3 Cups Peaches, fresh or frozen, peeled, sliced and thawed
1/2 Cup Blueberries, fresh or frozen, thawed
2 Tablespoons Honey

Glaze:
1 teaspoon Honey
1 Tablespoon Water

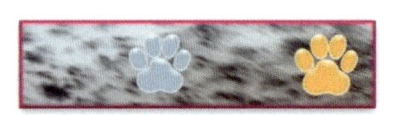

In the medium bowl, combine crust ingredients. Add more water if necessary to make a soft dough that sticks together. Let dough rest in bowl for 15-30 minutes.

In the small bowl, combine peaches, blueberries, and honey.

Cut parchment paper to fit baking sheet. Using a rolling pin, roll dough into a 12-inch circle on the parchment paper.

Place the peach mixture in the center of the dough circle leaving a 3-inch border.

Fold edges of dough toward center over peach mixture, pressing gently to seal. The dough will partially cover the peach mixture.

Mix the honey and water in a small cup. Brush over crust edges and peach mixture.

Bake at 450 Degrees for 10 minutes.

Reduce oven to 350 Degrees and bake for 20 more minutes until lightly browned.

Cool on wire rack.

SERVING SIZE:
Makes 8 servings
Serving size: 1 slice
Calories per serving: 230

Human: 1 serving
Canine:
Extra Large: 3/4 serving
Large: 1/2 serving
Medium: 1/4 serving
Small: 1/8 serving

SERVING SUGGESTIONS:
Serve warm with a dollop of "I'm Whupped" Cream (Page 118).

TIPS:
Vary your fruit combinations to mix it up.

Try canola oil in your crust and replace 1/4 cup of the hard white wheat flour with almond, coconut, or quinoa flour for a different taste or texture.

Eat Your Own Dog Food Series

Coconut MacaLunas

4-PAWS
We love coconut. Be sure to beat the egg whites until stiff and don't overbake. These become moist and chewy the next day.

OVEN: 350 Degrees F
EQUIPMENT: Medium Bowl, Electric Mixer, Baking Sheet, Parchment Paper

6 Egg whites
1/4 teaspoon salt
1/2 Cup Agave Nectar
1 Tablespoon Vanilla
3 Cups Unsweetened
  Shredded Coconut

In the medium mixing bowl, beat egg whites and salt with electric mixer until stiff.

With a large spoon, fold in agave, vanilla, and coconut.

Line a baking sheet with parchment paper. Drop batter onto parchment paper, one rounded Tablespoon at a time.

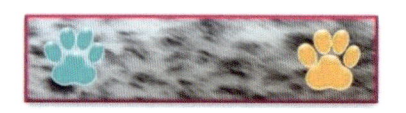

Bake for 10-15 minutes until lightly browned.

SERVING SIZE:
Makes 48 cookies
Serving size: 4 cookies
Calories per serving: 112

Human: 1 serving
Canine:
Extra Large: 1/2 serving
Large: 1/2 serving
Medium: 1/4 serving
Small: 1/8 - 1/4 serving

Rice Pudding with Dates

4-PAWS
Quick and easy, packed with complex carbohydrates and protein. Reminds you of your grandma's rice pudding, but a lot quicker to make.

OVEN: N/A
EQUIPMENT: Medium Saucepan.

2 Cups **Cooked** Brown Rice
2 Cups Lowfat Milk
1/4 Cup Honey
1/2 Cup Chopped Dried Dates
1 teaspoon Vanilla Extract
2 Large Eggs, beaten
2 Tablespoons Heavy Whipping Cream (optional)

___

In a medium saucepan, combine cooked rice, milk, honey, and dates. Heat over medium heat until mixture beings to simmer.

Reduce heat and simmer for about 5 minutes, stirring often to prevent burning.

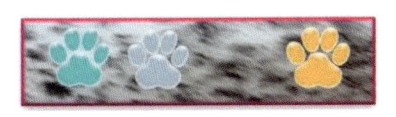

Stir in vanilla extract, eggs, and whipping cream.

Simmer 2-3 more minutes. Serve warm in a bowl.

SERVING SIZE:
Makes 6 servings
Serving size: 1/2 cup
Calories per serving: 220

Human: 1 serving
Canine:
Extra Large: 1 serving
Large: 1 serving
Medium: 1/2 serving
Small: 1/8 - 1/4 serving

Cabbage Carrot Cake with Honey Cream Cheese

4-PAWS
A spin on traditional carrot cake you will love with a little dab of cream cheese topping.

OVEN: 350 Degrees F
EQUIPMENT: Large Bowl, Electric Mixer, 2 9-inch Round Cake Pans or 13 x 9 Baking Pan

2 1/4 Cups Hard White Wheat Flour
2 teaspoons Baking Soda
1 teaspoon Baking Powder
2 teaspoons Cinnamon
1/4 teaspoon Nutmeg
3/4 Cup Honey
3 Large Eggs
3/4 Cup Buttermilk
1 Cup Canola Oil
3 teaspoons Vanilla Extract
1 Cup Nonfat Yogurt
3/4 Cup Shredded Carrots
3/4 Cup Shredded Red Cabbage
3/4 Cup Pecans, chopped
Nonstick Cooking Spray
1 8-ounce package of Cream Cheese, softened
3 Tablespoons Honey

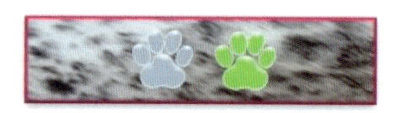

Preheat the oven and spray pan(s) with nonstick cooking spray.

In a medium bowl, combine flour, baking soda, baking powder, cinnamon, and nutmeg.

Add honey, eggs, buttermilk, oil, vanilla extract, and yogurt to dry ingredients and mix using the electric mixer on medium-high until smooth.

Using a spoon, fold in carrots, cabbage, and pecans. Mix well.

Pour into prepared pans and bake 25-35 minutes until done and a toothpick inserted in center comes out clean.

Let stand in pans for 10 minutes. Turn out on wire cooling rack to cool completely.

With an electric mixer, whip cream cheese and honey until smooth.

Spread on top(s) of the cake(s). Stack layers if desired, sprinkle with chopped pecans.

SERVING SIZE:
Makes 16 servings
Serving size: 1 slice
Calories per serving: 335

Human: 1 serving
Canine:
Extra Large: 1 serving
Large: 1 serving
Medium: 1/2 serving
Small: 1/8 - 1/4 serving

SERVING SUGGESTIONS:
Serve warm or chilled.

TIPS:
The honey adds a slight sweetness to the cream cheese without all the sugar in traditional cream cheese frosting.

Eat Your Own Dog Food Series

Lip-Licking-Lemon Cheesecake Bites

4-PAWS
Great lemony flavor and a great source of calcium and phosphorus. The honey adds just a hint of sweetness.

OVEN: 325 Degrees F
EQUIPMENT: 12-Cup Muffin Pan, Muffin Liners, Small and Medium Bowls, Electric Mixer or Stick Blender

Crust:
1 Cup Almond Flour
3 Tablespoons Honey
3 Tablespoons Melted Butter

Filling:
1 8-ounce Package Lowfat Cream Cheese, softened
1/4 Cup Honey
2 Tablespoons Whole Wheat Flour
1 Tablespoon Lemon Juice
2 teaspoons Lemon Rind
1/4 teaspoon Vanilla Extract
2 Large Eggs

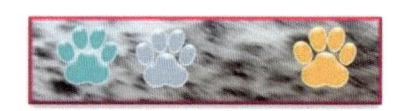

Preheat the oven. Line each muffin cup.

Combine flour, honey, and butter to form crust. Split crust mixture evenly in the 12 muffin liners and press lightly to form a bottom crust in each cup.

Combine all filling ingredients. Mix at medium speed until well blended and smooth.

Pour mixture over crust in each cup dividing evenly in the 12 cups.

Bake for 25 minutes until filling is set.

Remove from pan and cool completely. Remove from liner before serving.

SERVING SIZE:
Makes 12 mini cakes
Serving size: 1 cake
Calories per serving: 185

Human: 1 serving
Canine:
Extra Large: 1 serving
Large: 3/4 serving
Medium: 1/2 serving
Small: 1/8 - 1/4 serving

SERVING SUGGESTIONS:
Serve chilled with a dollop of "I'm Whupped" Cream (Page 118).

TIPS:
Try other citrus flavors and fruit purées to make these tasty little treats.

Be careful, these can be addicting.

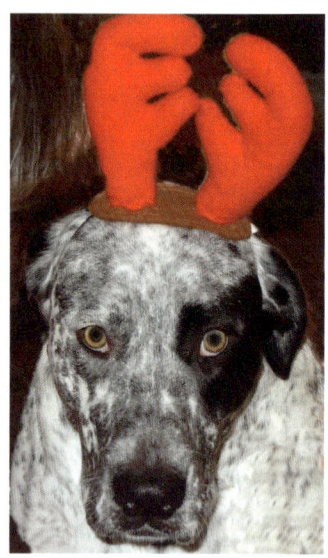

"I know, don't say it..."

Special Theme-Day ARF-Fairs

One day a month, my mom plans a special theme-day that we enjoy together. Here are a few of my favorite combinations. I can hardly wait until dessert time!

All of these recipes are included in the prior sections. Have your parents mix and match to create their own special theme-days for your family.

If you have questions about any recipe contained in this book, please email your questions to us at **eatwithluna@gmail.com**.

Receive new recipes and theme-day ideas each week by joining our online community at
www.eatyourowndogfood.net

1. **Happy BARKday Bash:** Garden Fettuccine ARFredo with Chicken, Pear and Candied Walnut Salad, and Cabbage Carrot Cake with Cream Cheese Frosting.

2. **Backyard BARKeque:** PAWed-Pork Sandwich, Cool-Slaw, and HOWL-wiian Shortcake with I'm Whupped Cream.

3. **Grande Blue Gascon Plate Special**: LenTAIL Pot Pie, Cauliflower-Carrot Mash, and Pear/Apple Galette with "I'm Whupped" Cream.

4. **SNOOPER-Bowl Sunday Party**: Grilled Buffalo Chicken Sliders, Sweet Potato Fries, Drunken Green Beans, and Banana-Custard Pie.

5. **ItailWAGGIN' Feast**: Beef and Vegetable Spaghetti, Parmesan-Zucchini Crisps, and Lemon Cheesecake Bites.

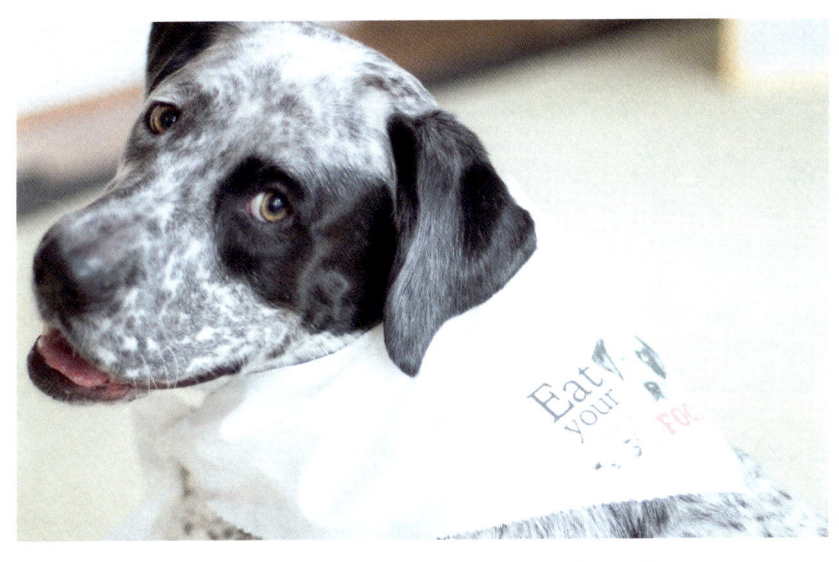

"Enough said, are you convinced yet?"

Appendix A: Pantry, Refrigerator, & Freezer Inventory

Pantry

Flours & Meals:
 Whole Grain Flour
 Hard White Wheat Flour
 Brown Rice Flour
 Almond Flour
 Coconut Flour
 Ground Flax seed
 Corn Meal
 Polenta

Rice, Grains, & Pasta:
 Whole Grain Brown Rice
 Brown Rice Pasta (various)
 Mixed Grains
 Rolled Oats
 Barley

Dried Beans & Legumes:
 Pinto
 Kidney
 Black
 Lima
 Garbanzo
 Navy
 Lentils
 Wheat Berries

Dried Fruits:
 Dates
 Cherries
 Apricots
 Figs

Nuts & Seeds:
 Almonds
 Pecans
 Walnuts
 Sunflower Seeds
 Sesame Seeds

Sweeteners:
 Honey
 Agave Nectar

Oils:
 Olive
 Canola
 Coconut
 Dark Sesame

Other:
 Sardines (in water or olive oil)
 Organic Tomato Paste (no sugar or salt added)
 Soy Sauce
 White Vinegar
 Apple Cider Vinegar
 Balsamic Vinegar
 Rice Wine Vinegar
 White Popcorn Kernels
 Peanut Butter (no sugar added)

Dry or Fresh Spices:
 Basil
 Black Pepper
 Cayenne Pepper
 Chili Powder

Pantry (cont.)

Cinnamon
Cloves
Cumin
Oregano
Italian Seasoning
Marjoram
Nutmeg
Ginger
Turmeric
Anise Seed
Fennel Seed
Cilantro
Parsley

Baking:
Baking Soda
Baking Powder
Salt
Yeast
Vanilla Extract
Nonfat Powdered Milk
Arrowroot
Cream of Tartar

Paper/Plastic Products:
Plastic Wrap
Aluminum Foil
Muffin Liners (paper)
Parchment Paper
Re-sealable Storage Bags:
 Sandwich
 One Quart
 One Gallon

Refrigerator

Lemon Juice
Lime Juice
Mustard
Yogurt
Milk
Heavy Whipping Cream
Eggs
Butter

Cheeses:
 Cottage
 Mozzarella
 Pecorino Romano
 Goat
 Cream Cheese
 Feta
 Gorgonzola

Fresh Fruits

Apples
Pears
Bananas
Blueberries
Strawberries
Watermelon
Honeydew
Cantaloupe
Plums
Peaches
Kiwi
Oranges
Tangerines
Lemons
Limes

Eat Your Own Dog Food Series

Fresh Vegetables

Tomatoes
Mushrooms
Green Peppers
Red, Yellow, Orange Peppers
Bok Choy
Kale
Collard Greens
Escarole (Endive)
Mustard Greens
Beet Greens
Romaine Lettuce
Yellow Squash
Zucchini Squash
Butternut Squash
Asparagus
Carrots
Spinach
Broccoli
Cauliflower
Celery
Sweet Potatoes
Parsnips
Beets
Red Cabbage
Green Cabbage

Freezer

Frozen Fruits:
 Blueberries
 Mixed Berries
 Peaches
 Strawberries

Frozen Vegetables:
 Green Beans
 Broccoli
 Mixed Vegetables
 Edamame
 Peas
 Corn
 Brussel Sprouts
 Artichoke Hearts

Appendix B: Other Tips & Suggestions

Homemade Broth
To make your own broth for soups and stews, add meat and spices or vegetables and spices to a large stockpot. Add enough water to cover the contents. Boil for 1 hour or until meat and/or vegetables are cooked.

Strain broth and skim off fat when cooled. For a quick method to remove fat from meat broths, strain the broth, place broth in the freezer for 2 hours. Fat hardens and can be removed easily. Portion broth into meal-sized containers and freeze for future use.

When precooking meats in the Electric Pressure Cooker, strain and skim off fat. Portion juices and use later for broth.

Fruit & Vegetable Purées
To make purées: core, peel, and cook fruit slightly in microwave safe container. Purée with a stick blender or food processor. For added nutrition, leave skin on.

Grains and Flours
These recipes use multigrain flours and specialty flours. Always use multigrain flour if you need to substitute for the almond, coconut, or quinoa flours.

PLUS Additions: Meat
Always have a supply of cooked beef, chicken, and pork on hand to add to your meals, and make extra meat when preparing your main meals.

PLUS Additions: Egg Shells
Store egg shells in the refrigerator in an air-tight container.

Vegetables & Greens
Don't be afraid to substitute other greens and change up vegetable combinations in the recipes.